Data Interpretation Questions and Case Histories
MRCP Part 2

D0243004

Biomedical Library

Queen's University Belfast

Tel: 028 9097 2710

E-mail: biomed.info@qub.ac.uk

For due dates and renewals:

QUB borrowers see 'MY ACCOUNT' at
http://library.qub.ac.uk/qcat
or go to the Library Home Page

HPSS borrowers see 'MY ACCOUNT' at
www.honni.qub.ac.uk/qcat

This book must be returned not later than its due
date, but is subject to recall if in demand

Fines are imposed on overdue books

Other books in The Complete MRCP series

Multiple Choice Questions
MRCP Part 1
H L C Beynon, C Marguerie, K Davies

Slide Interpretation Questions
MRCP Part 2
H L C Beynon, C Marguerie, C Craddock

With contributions to this volume by
A J Bishop MA MRCP
Registrar in Medicine
Hammersmith Hospital
London

M K B Whyte BSc MRCP
Registrar in Medicine
Hammersmith Hospital
London

H Thomas MA MRCP
Registrar in Clinical Oncology
Hammersmith Hospital
London

For Churchill Livingstone:

Publisher: Laurence Hunter
Editorial Co-ordination: Editorial Resources Unit
Production Controller: Mrs N G C Small
Design: Design Resources Unit
Sales Promotion Executive: Marion Pollock

Data Interpretation Questions and Case Histories
MRCP Part 2

H L C Beynon BSc MRCP
Registrar in Medicine
Royal Postgraduate Medical School
Hammersmith Hospital
London

C Marguerie BSc MRCP
Registrar in Medicine
Royal Postgraduate Medical School
Hammersmith Hospital
London

K A Davies MA MRCP
Senior Registrar
Department of Rheumatology
Royal Postgraduate Medical School
Hammersmith Hospital
London

C N Ross MRCP
Senior Registrar in Renal Medicine
Royal Postgraduate Medical School
Hammersmith Hospital
London

C Craddock BM BCh MRCP
Registrar in Haematology
Royal Postgraduate Medical School
Hammersmith Hospital
London

Foreword by
Mark J Walport MA PhD FRCP
Reader in Rheumatology, Department of Medicine,
Hammersmith Hospital, London

CHURCHILL
LIVINGSTONE

EDINBURGH LONDON MELBOURNE NEW YORK AND TOKYO 1991

CHURCHILL LIVINGSTONE
Medical Division of Pearson Professional Ltd.

Distributed in the United States of America by Churchill Livingstone Inc.,
650 Avenue of the Americas, New York, N. Y. 10011, and by associated
companies, branches and representatives throughout the world.

First published 1991
    Reprinted 1993
    Reprinted 1994
    Reprinted 1995
    Reprinted 1996
    Reprinted 1997

ISBN 0-443-04310-8

British Library Cataloguing in Publication Data
CIP catalogue record for this book is available from the British Library.

Library of Congress Cataloging in Publication Data
Data interpretation questions and case histories : MRCP part 2/
    H. L. C. Beynon . . . [et al.]; foreword by Mark J. Walport.
    p. cm.- (Complete MRCP series)
    Includes bibliographical references and index.
    1. Diagnosis - Examinations, questions, etc. 2. Diagnosis - Case
    studies.   I. Beynon, H. L. C.   II. Series
    [DNLM: 1. Diagnosis - case studeis. 2. Diagnosis - examination
    questions. 3. Disease - examination questions. WB 18 D232]
    RC71.3.D37   1991
    616.07′5′078-dc20
    DNLM/DLC
    for Library of Congress   91-8295
                                                                    CIP

Produced by Longman Singapore Publishers (Pte) Ltd
Printed in Singapore

Foreword to The Complete MRCP

The MRCP examination aims to test a broad range of clinical skills and background knowledge at an early stage of training in general medicine. The Part 1 examination provides an assessment of general medical knowledge and the written Part 2 assesses the ability to interpret clinical data and to identify those physical signs that can readily be photographed.

The format of the examination is influenced by the large number of candidates and the necessity to provide a test of uniform standard. Multiple choice questions (MCQs) provide a standardized assessment of knowledge. Studies conducted in disciplines other than medicine have shown that MCQs provide a discriminator of abilities that correlates with other tests such as the writing of essays. Animated discussion of the answers to multiple choice questions posed in the examination often engenders paranoia about the ambiguity or idiocy of particular questions. In reality, the answers to clinical questions are rarely black and white, as demanded by MCQs. However, the occasional obscure or ambiguous question that slips into the exam will be detected during marking of the papers and will not be used again. Such questions will only damage individual candidates if the fury they engender at the time disturbs a balanced approach to answering the remainder of the questions. The 'grey' cases and slide questions provide tests that approximate more closely to the reality of the bedside and probe comprehension of relevant clinical physiology and pathology.

This series of three books has been written by junior doctors who have not yet forgotten the agonies of the MRCP examination and who participate actively in teaching others who are about to confront the same hurdle. These books provide stimulating examples of the types of question encountered in all three sections of the MRCP examination, and provide an entertaining and informative journey through many of the highways and byways of medicine.

London 1991

M. J. W.

Preface

This is the second book in the series 'The Complete MRCP' and is complementary to Books 1 and 3. Book 1 contains 250 MCQs with expanded answers and covers Part 1 of the MRCP. Book 3 covers the projected material section.

Book 2 contains a selection of data interpretation questions and case histories similar to that encountered in Part 2 of the MRCP examination.

Where relevant many of the questions are accompanied by expanded answers to aid revision. We strongly recommend that candidates familiarise themselves with the sample exam questions published by the Royal College of Physicians; in the exam, concise simple answers are required and the college booklet is illuminating in this respect.

We hope this series will be both stimulating and helpful for candidates preparing for the examination.

1991   H. L. C. Beynon

Contents

Table of normal values

Urea, electrolytes and liver function tests

Sodium	136–149 mmol/l
Potassium	3.8–5 mmol/l
Bicarbonate	24–30 mmol/l
Urea	2.5–6.5 mmol/l
Chloride	93–108 mmol/l
Creatinine	55–125 µmol/l
Total Protein	65–80 g/l
Albumin	35–55 g/l
Calcium	2.15–2.65 mmol/l
Phosphate	0.80–1.4 mmol/l
Bilirubin	2–13 µmol/l
Alkaline phosphatase	30–130 iu/l
Aspartate amino-transferase	5–27 iu/l
Uric acid	0.1–0.4 mmol/l
Gamma GT	0–30 iu/l
Creatinine kinase	0–170 iu/l
Plasma Osmolality	285–295 mosmol/Kg

Miscellaneous

Cholesterol	3.6–7.2 mmol/l
Triglyceride	0–1.5 mmol/l
Glucose	3.5–5.5 mmol/l
Immunoglobulins	
IgG	5–16 g/l
IgA	1.25–4.25 g/l
IgM	0.5–1.7 g/l
C-reactive protein	0–10 mg/l
Iron	
males	16–30 µmol/l
females	11–27 µmol/l
Total iron binding capacity	45–72 µmol/l
Vitamin B_{12}	200–900 pg/ml
Serum folate	1.8–14 µg/l
Magnesium	0.65–1 mmol/l
Fecal fat excretion	11–18 mmol/l

Hormone levels

Cortisol	
9 am	170–720 nmol/l
midnight	170–220 nmol/l
Growth hormone	<10 ng/ml
Thyroxine	70–160 nmol/l
Thyroid-stimulating hormone	0.8–3.6 mU/l

Haematology

Haemoglobin	
males	13.5–17.5 g/dl
females	11.5–15.5 g/dl
Red blood cell count	
males	$4.5–6.5 \times 10^{12}/l$
females	$3.9–5.6 \times 10^{12}/l$
Packed cell volume	
males	0.4–0.54 l/l
females	0.35–0.47 l/l
Mean corpuscular haemoglobin	27–32 pg
Mean corpuscular haemoglobin concentration	32–36 g/dl
Mean corpuscular volume	76–98 fl
Reticulocyte count	0.2–2%
Platelet count	$150–400 \times 10^9/l$
White blood count	$4–11 \times 10^9/l$
Neutrophils	$2.5–7.58 \times 10^9/l$
Lymphocytes	$1.5–3.5 \times 10^9/l$
Eosinophils	$0.04–0.44 \times 10^9/l$
Basophils	$0–0.1 \times 10^9/l$
Monocytes	$0.2–0.8 \times 10^9/l$
Erythrocyte sedimentation rate	0–10 mm in the first hour
Prothrombin time	12–15.5 sec
Activated partial thromboplastin time	30–46 sec
Thrombin time	15–19 sec
Bleeding time	2–8 mins
Fibrinogen	2–4 g/l

Cardiology normal values

	Mean (mmHg)	Range (mmHg)
R.A.	4	0–8
R.V.		
systolic	25	15–30
end diastolic	4	0–8
P.A.P.		
systolic	25	15–30
diastolic	10	5–15
mean	15	10–20
P.A.W.P.	10	5–14
L.V.		
systolic	120	90–140
end diastolic	7	4–12
Aorta		
systolic	120	90–140
diastolic	70	60–90
mean	85	70–105

Questions

1 A 60 year old woman was brought to casualty unconscious. Her blood glucose was 2.6 mmol/l. She was resuscitated with intravenous glucose. She gave a 3-month history of early morning dizziness. Past medical history was unremarkable.

Investigations:

Fasting blood glucose   2.7 mmol/l
Blood insulin   16 mU/l
Hb 14 g/dl MCV   84 fl
Urea/electrolytes/liver function tests normal

a) What is the diagnosis?
b) What is the differential diagnosis and how would you distinguish between them?

2 A You are asked to see a diabetic patient preoperatively because of the following electrolytes.

Sodium   123 mmol/l
Potassium   2.9 mol/l
Urea   4 mmol/l
Glucose,   47 mmol/l
Bicarbonate   19 mmol/l

a) What is the likely explanation?

B You receive the following report; the blood was drawn on the previous evening.

Sodium   136 mmol/l
Potassium   9 mmol/l
Urea   14 mol/l
Creatinine   220 µmol/l
Glucose   1.6 mmol/l
Phosphate   3.8 mmol/l
Calcium   2.1 mmol/l

a) What is likely explanation?

C

	Sample 1	Sample 2
Albumin	40 g/l	43 g/l
Calcium	2.28 mmol/l	2.41 mmol/l
Haemoglobin	14 g/dl	14.9 g/dl
Potassium	3.8 mmol/l	3.7 mmol/l

a) How do you account for the disparity between the two sets of blood results taken on the same patient 20 minutes apart?

3 This patient presented with recurrent collapse. She was on no drugs.

12.5 mm/sec; 0.5 cm/mV

a) What is the likely underlying disease?
b) What treatment will be required?
c) What is the theoretical danger of atrioversion with quinidine?

Question 4

4 A 32 year old non-smoker is admitted for investigation and treatment of severe shortness of breath. The following results are obtained:

Hb	14.3 g/dl
WCC	15.4 $\times 10^9$/l
Neutrophils	74%
Lymphocytes	12%
Eosinophils	11%
pO_2	8.4 kPa
pCO_2	5.4 kPa
PEFR	80 l/sec
Flow–volume loop	A

The patient's condition deteriorates over the next 12 hours and he is subsequently electively ventilated via a cuffed endotracheal tube. He is weaned from the ventilator 4 weeks later. A flow–volume loop is performed 4 months later (B).

a) What diagnosis would account for i) the first and ii) the second flow–volume loops?

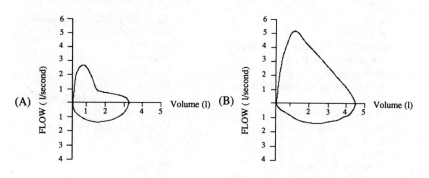

5 A 10 year old Asian girl attended hospital complaining of a 10-day history of fever and malaise. Her ankles, right wrist and left knee had been stiff and painful for 5 days. Her general practitioner had seen her 2 weeks previously and given her a course of antibiotics for a sore throat and mild upper respiratory tract infection. She was treated with aspirin, following which her fever settled over 48 hours and her joints became much less painful.

She had no previous history of joint problems. Twelve weeks before she had returned from a 6-week holiday in Pakistan, where both she and her brother had contracted hepatitis. She had received primary chemoprophylaxis for tuberculosis at the age of nine.

Examination
Temperature 39°C, no pharyngitis, no lymphadenopathy, no skin rashes. Pulse 90 regular, JVP not elevated, normal first and second heart sounds and a soft pericardial rub. She had no hepatosplenomegaly. The painful joints were swollen.

Investigations:

Hb	10 g/l
MCV	80 fl
WBC	12 × 10^9/l 70% neutrophils
Platelets	400 × 10^9/l.
Haemoglobin electrophoresis	normal
Urea and electrolytes	normal
Bilirubin	7 μmol/l
Aspartate amino-transferase	65 iu/l
ESR	115 mm in the first hour
Latex and autoantibody screen	negative
Ig G	25 g/l
Ig A	3.14 g/l
Ig M	2.11 g/l
C-reactive protein	80 mg/l
Cultures of blood, urine and throat	negative
Paul–Bunnell	negative
Hepatitis B Ag	negative

Hepatitis A antibodies – acute serum 1/1280
– convalescent serum 1/640
ASO titre 500 iu/l acute serum, 800 iu/l convalescent
Left knee aspirate 20 mls of yellow fluid containing 3000 neutrophils/ml, sterile on culture
Urinalysis a trace of protein but no casts or cells on microscopy
CXR NAD, X-rays of the affected joints NAD
ECG sinus rhythm, PR interval 0.3 ms, normal axis, normal QRS
Echocardiogram – mild mitral regurgitation, small pericardial effusion

a) What is the most likely diagnosis?

b) What treatment would you give?

6A A middle-aged woman was referred with thirst, polydipsia and polyuria. She had been involved in a road traffic accident 9 months before and thought her symptoms had begun soon after this. She had no serious illness in the past and took no medication. General examination was normal B.P. 120/80 no postural drop. Her 24-hour urine collections were between 7 and 12 litres.

Investigations:

Sodium	130 mmol/l
Potassium	3.5 mmol/l
Urea	2.0 mmol/l
Glucose	5 mmol/l
Protein	70 g/l
Albumin	35 g/l
Alkaline phosphatase	80 iu/l
Bilirubin	5 μmol/l
Plasma osmolality	268 mosmol/l
Urine osmolality	50 mmol/l

a) What is the likely diagnosis?

b) What investigation would you arrange?

6B A 24 year old army private was admitted with a 24-hour history of coughing up bright red blood, and haematuria. On examination he was slightly agitated, temperature 37.2°C, pulse 100 and regular. Chest was clear to auscultation.

Investigations:

Hb	13.6 g/dl
WBC	$7 \times 10^9/l$
Platelets	$278 \times 10^9/l$
ESR	8 mm in the first hour
Urea	4 mmol/l
Chest X-ray	normal
Urine dipstick	protein ++, blood +++
Urine microscopy	100 RBC per high powered field numerous epithelial cells Gram positive cocci, gram positive rods, fusiform bacilli

a) What one diagnostic test would you perform to confirm your diagnosis?

7A A 65 year old lady with disseminated carcinoma of the ovary is admitted for a further course of chemotherapy. Four days after admission she complains of perioral paraesthesia.

Investigations:

Sodium	137 mmol/l
Potassium	4 mmol/l
Bicarbonate	26 mmol/l
Urea	5 mmol/l
Creatinine	120 µmol/l
Calcium	1.6 mmol/l
Phosphate	1.20 mmol/l
Albumin	37 g/l
Alkaline phosphatase	110 iu/l

a) What two signs would you attempt to elicit?

b) What is the underlying biochemical abnormality, what is its origin and how should the patient be treated?

7B A 65 year old man is admitted through casualty with marked shortness of breath. On examination he is in atrial fibrillation with a radial rate of 145 and an apical–radial deficit of 30, blood pressure 148/92 mmHg, JVP elevated at 8 cm, cardiomegaly, gallop rhythm and an apical pansystolic murmur. Both lung bases are dull to percussion and there are end-inspiratory crepitations to the mid zones. Gross pitting ankle oedema to the mid thighs is present. On admission he is taking no regular medication.

Investigations:

Sodium	128 mmol/l
Potassium	2.9 mmol/l
Bicarbonate	30 mmol/l
Urea	8 mmol/l
Albumin	24 g/l
Bilirubin	43 µmol/l
Alkaline phosphatase	601 iu/l
Aspartate amino-transferase	40 iu/l
Chest X-ray	upper lobe blood diversion, alveolar oedema and bilateral effusions

a) What is the diagnosis?

b) How do you explain the biochemical abnormalities?

8 A 30 year old car mechanic presented to a follow-up clinic with an 8-week history of night sweats sufficient to soak the sheets, and right upper quadrant pain. He has lost 6 kg in 3 months and was drinking 2 pints of beer daily. On examination he was pyrexial 38.3°C, thin and pale with four-fingers' breadth of tender hepatomegaly. He had no lymphadenopathy and was not icteric.

Past medical history: Hodgkin's disease stage III diagnosed 1 year previously, treated with combined chemotherapy.

Investigations:

Hb	11.8 g/dl
WBC	2.4 × 10⁹/l–70% neutrophils
Platelets	345 × 10⁹/l
Sodium	139 mmol/l
Potassium	4.5 mmol/l
Bicarbonate	27 mmol/l
Creatinine	87 μmol/l
Alkaline phosphatase	372 iu/l
Aspartate transaminase	79 iu/l
Bilirubin	24 μmol/l
Albumin	36 g/l
Protein	72 g/l
CXR	diffuse bilateral infiltration with occasional nodules.

a) List 3 possible causes of this clinical picture

b) List 3 important diagnostic procedures

9 An 11 year old girl presents with a 4-hour history of passing fresh blood per rectum. Past medical history is unremarkable. Earlier that day she had played a 2-hour game of tennis. She is on no regular medication and there is no significant family history. On examination she has a regular pulse of 120 and a blood pressure of 100/65 mmHg supine and 80/55 mmHg erect. Oral mucosa is normal. The abdomen is soft and there is no organomegaly. Rectal examination and sigmoidoscopy reveal normal perianal skin and normal rectal mucosa.

Investigations:

Hb	12 g/dl
MCV	83 fl
WBC	5 × 10⁹/l
Platelets	240 × 10⁹/l
PT	12 s
PTTK	36 s
Urea and electrolytes	normal
Chest X-ray	normal

The patient is resuscitated. An emergency gastroscopy is performed which shows normal stomach and duodenum.

a) What is the likely diagnosis?

b) How would you confirm your diagnosis?

10 A 50 year old man is admitted for investigation of recurrent peptic ulceration. His problems first started at 43 years of age when he was resident in Delhi and was admitted for emergency surgery to repair a perforated peptic ulcer. Three years later he underwent a Polya partial gastrectomy for recurrent peptic ulceration. Since this time he has been persistently troubled by abdominal pain worse at night and diarrhoea with 4 loose motions a day. His current medication is ranitidine 150 mg b.d. together with liberal doses of antacids.

Investigations:

Hb	10 g/dl
MCV	76 fl
MCH	26 pg
MCHC	30 g/dl
Urea and electrolytes	normal
Liver function tests	normal
Fasting serum gastrin	390 pmol/l (Normal <100 pmol/l)

Secretin test – intravenously 2 units GIH secretin per kg

Basal fasting	value	401 pmol/l
	10 min	265 pmol/l
	20 min	280 pmol/l
	30 min	300 pmol/l

a) What is the diagnosis?

b) How would you confirm your diagnosis?

11 A 40 year old Chinese man, who was otherwise fit and well, was admitted for a hernia repair. He had lived and worked in the UK for 25 years. He drank no alcohol and took no herbal remedies or other medications. He had no history of illness in the past and had never had a blood transfusion. The following blood results were obtained:

Sodium	140 mmol/l
Potassium	4.0 mmol/l
Urea	6 mmol/l
Albumin	40 mg/l
AST	120 iu/l
ALP	140 iu/l
Bilirubin	10 μmol/l
HBs Ag	negative
HBê Ab	positive
ANA	negative
Latex	negative

a) What is the likely diagnosis?

b) What further investigations does this man require?

c) What are the indications for treatment of this condition?

Question 12

12 A 77 year old man presented to outpatients complaining of weakness in both legs. Over the previous 3 months he had felt listless and had lost 5 kg in weight. He had suffered from lumbar spondylosis for several years; 4 months ago he developed upper and mid back pain which had recently radiated round to his umbilicus and required regular codeine phosphate. Two weeks previously he had developed a mild fever and night sweats and had been given a short course of antibiotics. On direct questioning he admitted that recently his bowel habit had changed and he had needed regular glycerol suppositories. He smoked 20 cigarettes per day and suffered from chronic bronchitis with frequent infective exacerbations. Medication included salbutamol inhaler, and oral aminophylline.

On examination the patient was cachectic, alert and orientated. Temperature 38°C. There was no lymphadenopathy, clubbing, anaemia or jaundice. Examination of his chest revealed a mild expiratory wheeze in both lung fields. Cardiovascular examination was normal. His cervical spine was normal, the lower 6 thoracic and all lumbar vertebrae were tender. The cranial nerves and fundi were normal. Hip and knee flexion was weak bilaterally; other muscle groups had normal strength. Light touch and pin prick were reduced in both lower limbs with a sensory level just below the umbilicus. Vibration sense and proprioception were reduced in both feet. The tendon reflexes were present and equal. The plantar reflexes were extensor on both sides. Rectal tone was normal, voluntary contraction intact, the prostate gland was smooth with a normal sulcus.

Investigations:

Hb	14 g/l
WBC	8 × 10⁹/l
Platelets	450 × 10⁹/l
ESR	17 mm in the first hour
Sodium	140 mmol/l
Potassium	4 mmol/l
Urea	6.5 mmol/l
CRP	10 mg/l
Aspartate amino-transferase	27 iu/l
Alkaline phosphatase	170 iu/l
Creatine phosphokinase	20 iu/l
Acid phosphatase	0.8 u/l (normal <3.3 u/l)

CXR lung fields clear, the 8th and 9th thoracic vertebrae were sclerotic and reduced in height; there was loss of the intervertebral disc space.
ECG sinus rhythm 76, normal axis

a) What is the most likely diagnosis?

b) What investigations would you request and what treatment would you advise?

13 A 12 year old boy is referred to outpatients with nocturnal enuresis. His mother comments that he is easily tired by sport and is not doing well at school. He is normotensive and on the 8th centile for height.

Investigations:

Sodium	145 mmol/l
Potassium	2.8 mmol/l
Bicarbonate	35 mmol/l
Chloride	80 mmol/l
Urea	5 mmol/l
Glucose	4.4 mmol/l
24 hour urine	60 mmol of potassium
	60 mmol of sodium

a) What is the likely diagnosis?

14 A 35 year old man is sectioned and admitted to the psychiatric ward with a diagnosis of acute schizophrenia. Six days later he becomes pyrexial and is unable to eat; his condition deteriorates over the next 24 hours and he becomes increasingly confused. On examination, positive findings were a temperature of 39.5°C, pulse of 130, blood pressure 145/90 mmHg, marked neck stiffness, normal fundi and symmetrically increased tone in all four limbs with flexor plantars.

Investigations:

Sodium	140 mmol/l
Potassium	4 mmol/l
Bicarbonate	28 mmol/l
Urea	5 mmol/l
Bilirubin	23 μmol/l
Alkaline phosphatase	120 iu/l
Aspartate amino-transferase	54 iu/l
Calcium	2.4 mmol/l
Creatinine kinase	980 iu/l
Glucose	4.3 mmol/l
Hb	12 g/dl
WBC	12×10^9/l
Platelets	230×10^9/l
Chest X-ray	normal
CT head	normal
CSF	
opening pressure	15 cm H2O
cell count	3 lymphocytes/mm³
protein	0.5 g/l
glucose	3 mmol/l
Blood cultures	sterile
Urine dipstick	negative blood, negative protein

a) What is the likely diagnosis?

15 A 44 year old man is admitted with a history of vomiting. He has been treated in the past for peptic ulceration and depression. He looks unwell, investigations show:

Hb	16.3 g/dl
WBC	11.1 × 10⁹/l
Platelets	354 × 10⁹/l
Sodium	138 mmol/l
Potassium	2.8 mmol/l
Urea	14.3 mmol/l
pH	7.52
pO₂	12.4 kPa
pCO₂	5.5 kPa
Bicarbonate	36 mmol/l
Chloride	75 mmol/l

a) What is the metabolic abnormality?
b) What is the likely diagnosis?
c) Would the patient's urine be acid or alkaline?
d) Explain the basis of the metabolic upset in this situation.

16A A 70 year old woman was admitted in congestive cardiac failure. Past medical history – treated hypertension for 5 years.

Investigations:

Hb	7.5 g/dl
WBC	6.5 × 10⁹/l
Platelets	235 × 10⁹/l
MCV	106 fl
Reticulocytes	24%
Bilirubin	40 μmol/l
Aspartate amino-transferase	25 iu/l
Alkaline phosphatase	120 iu/l

a) What is the likely diagnosis?
b) What further investigation would you order?

16B A 25 year old woman becomes unwell with fever, sore throat and dysphagia. On examination she has a temperature of 38°C, a fine tremor and a diffusely tender thyroid gland.

Investigations:

Hb	14 g/dl
WBC	6 × 10⁹/l
ESR	65 mm in the first hour
T4	190 nmol/l
⁹⁹Tc-isotope scan	no uptake

a) What is the diagnosis?
b) How would you treat her?

17 A 69 year old man presents to his GP with a 4-month history of progressive weakness, and difficulty with swallowing and mastication. Examination reveals widespread wasting and fasciculation in upper and lower limbs, a wasted fasciculating tongue and a left partial ptosis.

a) Name two possible diagnoses, in order of likelihood.

b) Which finding makes one diagnosis more likely?

c) What investigations would you perform to distinguish these two possibilities?

18 A 56 year old doctor returned to the UK after a 5-week holiday in Malaysia. He had an unremarkable past medical history and had been well up until 18 months previously when he started to complain of general lethargy. Over the past 4 months he lost 4.5 kg in weight and had developed low backache and intermittent diarrhoea. On average he smoked 25 cigarettes and drank 3 pints of beer each day. On examination he was suntanned, clinically anaemic and had several small nodes palpable in the axillae. Abdominal examination was normal. He was weak proximally but all reflexes were present and symmetrical. Mild pitting oedema was present.

Investigations:

Hb	10 g/dl
MCV	101 fl
MCHC	32 g/dl
WBC	5×10^9/l
Platelets	260×10^9/l
Urea	4 mmol/l
Creatinine	105 µmol/l
Sodium	135 mmol/l
Potassium	3.8 mmol/l
Albumin	28 g/l
Calcium	1.8 mmol/l
Phosphate	0.7 mmol/l
Alkaline phosphatase	188 iu/l
Bilirubin	17 µmol/l
Aspartate amino-transferase	25 iu/l
Faecal fat excretion	>26 mmol/l

a) What is the most likely diagnosis? How do you explain the neurological signs present?

b) How would you confirm your diagnosis?

c) What treatment would you institute?

19 This is the M-mode echocardiogram of a 17 year old boy who faints with exercise.

a) Comment on structures A and B.

b) What is the pathophysiological significance of space C, and how will it be affected by squatting?

c) Give two reasons for the exertional syncope.

20 A 38 year old lorry driver was referred with a rash presumed to be secondary to amoxycillin. He had presented to his GP 5 days before with a 6-day history of anorexia, fever and headache, and a 3-day history of dry cough and mild dyspnoea. He has no chest pain or haemoptysis. He smoked 10 cigarettes per day and drank 3–4 pints of beer per day. He had had no serious illness in the past. He had been commenced on amoxycillin 500 mg t.d.s.

Examination: temperature 39°C, pulse 90, blood pressure 110/60. There was no clinical jaundice, anaemia, cyanosis or clubbing. Several fine crepitations could be heard in the right base. Over his trunk and upper arms he had a fine maculopapular rash; several target lesions were present. Otherwise general examination was normal. He was admitted to hospital.

Investigations:

Hb	13 g/dl
WBC	$10 \times 10^9/l$
Sodium	142 mmol/l
Potassium	4.4 mmol/l
Urea	9 mmol/l
Creatinine	90 μmol/l
ESR	70 cm in the first hour
Aspartate transaminase	90 iu/l
Alkaline phosphatase	150 iu/l
Bilirubin	12 μmol/l
Blood and sputum culture	negative
Cold agglutinins	positive
CXR	patchy consolidation right base.

Five days after admission the patient developed increasing fatigue, dyspnoea, palpitations, dull central chest pain and myalgia.

Examination: pulse 120, blood pressure 110/60. Chest signs unchanged. Heart sounds: first and second sounds normal plus a soft third heart sound.

Blood gases	pO_2 14 kPa pCO_2 5 kPa
CXR	no change
ECG	sinus tachycardia, widespread T-wave flattening and inversion.

Echocardiography showed normal valves and chambers. Contraction of the left ventricle was reduced.

a) Suggest a unifying diagnosis.

b) What further investigations would you arrange?

21 An 18 year old man, previously fit and on no medication becomes unwell with fever, myalgia, mild neck stiffness and loss of appetite. His GP diagnoses influenza. On review 48 hours later he is concerned that the patient is now clinically jaundiced and refers him to casualty.

Investigations:

Hb	14.8 g/dl
MCV	88 fl
Reticulocytes	1%
WBC	6×10^9/l
Platelets	259×10^9/l
ESR	10 cm in the first hour
Bilirubin	55 µmol/l
Conjugated bilirubin	9 µmol/l
Aspartate aminotransferase	25 iu/l
Alkaline phosphatase	105 iu/l
Albumin	42 g/l
Urea and electrolytes	normal

a) What is the likely diagnosis?

22 A 42 year old epileptic is admitted through casualty having been found unconscious at home. The following results are obtained 24 hours later:

Sodium	135 mmol/l
Potassium	6.7 mmol/l
Urea	18 mmol/l
Creatinine	630 µmol/l
Calcium	1.84 mmol/l
Aspartate amino-transferase	86 iu/l
Gamma-glutamyl transpeptidase	70 iu/l
Urine dipstick	blood ++
Ammonium sulphate test	coloured supernatant
Red cell transketolase	low

a) What condition do these results suggest?
b) Suggest 2 possible causes in this patient.

23 The following results are obtained in a 32 year old woman with a blood pressure of 184/114 mmHg.

Investigations:

Sodium	135 mmol/l
Potassium	5.2 mmol/l
Urea	11.2 mmol/l
Creatinine	212 µmol/l
Albumin	30 g/l
Urinalysis	Blood non-haemolysed trace Protein 5.4g/24 h
Urine microscopy	Scanty red cells and granular casts
HbA1c	3.4%
ANA	1:320 speckled pattern
Renal biopsy	Immunofluorescence: Linear IgG on glomerular basement membrane

a) What is the diagnosis?

b) What histological pattern is likely to be present in the kidney?

c) What is the likely course of the disease?

24 A 65 year old man is referred with glycosuria by his GP. He was asymptomatic, and on no regular medication. Six years ago he underwent surgery for a recurrent peptic ulcer.

A standard glucose tolerance test was performed.

Time	Blood glucose (venous) mmol/l	
0	4.8	No glycosuria
30 mins	12.5	
60 mins	9.8	Glycosuria
90 mins	2.3	
120 mins	3.2	

a) What does this investigation show?

b) What is the likely explanation in this case?

Question 25

25 A 32 year old woman presented with jaundice 2 months after
starting the oral contraceptive pill and 1 month after returning
from Turkey, where she had contracted a short-lived illness,
characterized by fever and diarrhoea. She had felt run down for
several months and attributed this to working long hours as a
barmaid. In Turkey, while sunbathing, she had noticed several
painless patches on her hands and face which did not tan. She
was on no regular medication. She was a non-smoker and
drank between 2 and 3 glasses of wine a day. On examination
there were depigmented areas on both hands and on her face.
She was icteric and several spider naevi was noted. Her heart,
lungs and abdomen were normal.

Investigations:

Hb	12 g/l
WBC	8 × 10⁹/l
Platelets	150 × 10⁹/l
MCV	99 fl
Bilirubin	90 μmol/l
Aspartate aminotransferase	185 iu/l
Alkaline phosphatase	200 iu/l
Total protein	80 g/l
Albumin	26 g/l
HBS Ag	negative
Hep A serology	positive 1/640
Rheumatoid factor	negative
ANA positive	1/160

a) What is the most likely diagnosis?

b) What three investigations would you request?

c) What immediate management steps would you take?

26 The patient has sustained an inferior myocardial infarction (ECG on facing page).

a) Which of the following drugs will exacerbate and which improve the problem demonstrated?

Digoxin	Verapamil
Isoprenaline	Adenosine
Atropine	Imipramine

27 A young woman presents with abdominal pain. The houseman shows you her electrolytes:

Sodium	134 mmol/l
Potassium	4.1 mmol/l
Bicarbonate	17 mmol/l
Urea	2.0 mmol/l
Creatinine	43 µmol/l
Total protein	72 g/l
Albumin	32 g/l
Calcium	2.14 mmol/l
Phosphate	1.23 mmol/l
Bilirubin	5 µmol/l
Alkaline phosphatase	400 iu/l
Aspartate aminotransferase	17 iu/l
Uric acid	0.1 mmol/l
Thyroxine	190 nmol/l

a) What is the underlying condition?

28 A 16 year old girl is reviewed 6-monthly, having been treated for acute lymphocytic leukaemia ten years previously. She has recently returned from Greece where she has been living for the past 2 years. She presents with a 6-month history of weight loss of 8 kg, general malaise and occasional fevers. Clinical examination is normal apart from signs of obvious weight loss.

Full blood count, urea, electrolytes and liver function tests are all normal.

a) Give three possible diagnoses and your reasons.

b) How would you exclude two of these with further investigations?

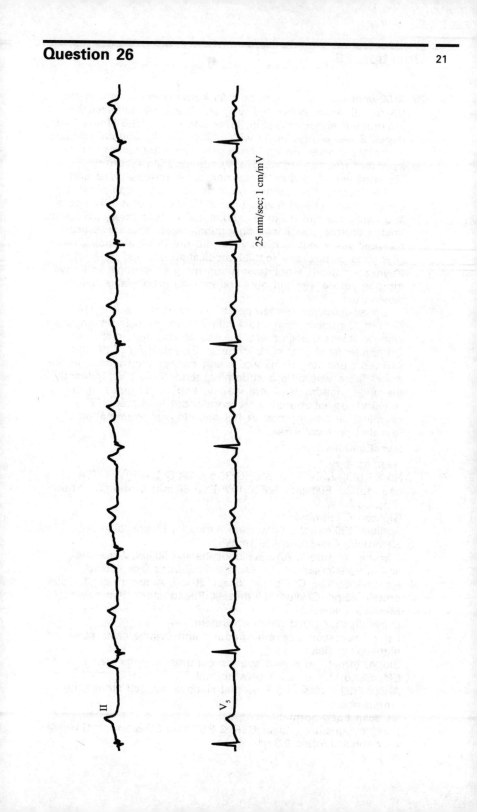

25 mm/sec; 1 cm/mV

II

V₅

29 A 30 year old Asian man, born in Kenya and resident in the UK for 15 years, presented with an illness characterized by intermittent abdominal pain, fever and rigors. The illness had begun 3 weeks previously with diffuse colicky abdominal pains and night sweats. He had been prescribed antibiotics and was symptom free for 3 days. His symptoms then recurred accompanied by a dull frontal headache, muscle pains and severe fatigue. For the last week he had had a non-productive cough, anorexia and fevers upto 39°C accompanied by rigors and chills. He had no other abdominal or respiratory symptoms apart from the cough and abdominal pains. There was no relevant past medical history. He did not drink alcohol, smoke cigarettes or take any regular medication. He had no foreign travel apart from a holiday visiting his grandparents in Kenya 2 months before. He had obtained malaria prophylaxis before leaving the UK.

On examination his temperature was 39.8°C, pulse 110, BP 110/60 mmHg, respiratory rate 20/min. He was lethargic and when disturbed, belligerent. He had no jaundice, rash, lymphadenopathy or neck stiffness. Examination of his chest showed clear lung fields and a soft pansystolic murmur at the apex. There was diffuse abdominal tenderness predominantly in the upper quadrants. There was no abdominal guarding or rebound. Bowel sounds were normal but infrequent. PR examination was normal. A full neurological examination revealed no focal signs.

Investigations:

Haematology:
Hb 8.5 g/dl, MCV 87 fl, MCHC 30 pg, WBC 7 × 10^9/l – 62% neutrophils, Platelets 128 × 10^9/l ESR 80 mm in the first hour.

Biochemistry:
Glucose 6.2 mmol/l
Sodium 130 mmol/l, Potassium 4 mmol/l, Bicarb 20 mmol/l, Urea 30 mmol/l, Creatinine 495 µmol/l.
Bilirubin 12 µmol/l, Alkaline phosphatase 50 iu/l, Aspartate amino-transferase 70 iu/l, Lactate dehydrogenase 495 iu/l, Amylase 60 iu/l, Creatinine kinase 50 iu/l, Albumin 28 g/l, Total protein 65 g/l, Calcium 1.7 mmol/l, Phosphate 1.19 mmol/l.

Miscellaneous:
Urine dipstick tests: blood +, protein +++
Urine microscopy: several granular and hyaline casts seen per high power field.
Blood, throat, urine and sputum cultures all negative.
Chest and abdominal X-rays normal
Abdominal ultrasound – normal kidneys, no gall stones, no lymph nodes
CT scan head normal.
Lumbar puncture – clear CSF, 2 RBC and 3WBC/mm³, Glucose 4.5 mmol/l, protein 0.3 g/l

a) What is the most likely diagnosis?
b) How would you confirm this?
c) What treatment would you give?

30 A 55 year old farmer complained of breathlessness and a dry cough which had worsened gradually over 3 months. Recently he had found working difficult because of dyspnoea and was considering retiring. He had occasional mild fevers and influenza-like symptoms and had lost 3 kg in weight over the past 2 months. Generally all of his symptoms were worse towards the end of the day. He had had an anterior myocardial infarct 5 years previously, complicated by left ventricular failure, now controlled with diuretics. He had had no further angina. He smoked 15 cigarettes daily until his myocardial infarction when on medical advice he had given up.

On examination there was no clubbing, anaemia, cyanosis, oedema or jaundice. The jugular venous pressure was normal, BP 150/70. Examination of his heart was unremarkable. On auscultation there were fine inspiratory crackles heard in both lung bases.

Investigations:

Hb	13.9 g/dl
WBC	$10 \times 10^9/l$
ESR	50 mm in the first hour
Sodium	137 mmol/l
Potassium	3.9 mmol/l
Urea	8 mmol/l
Albumin	43 g/l
Total protein	78 g/l
Aspartate transaminase	35 iu/l
Alkaline phosphatase	111 iu/l
Bilirubin	12 µmol/l
Latex	negative
ANA	negative

ECG showed the previous anterior myocardial infarction, but was otherwise unremarkable. A chest X-ray showed areas of nodular shadowing in both lung bases.

FEV1 70%; FVC 80%, VA 110%, DLCO to 70%, KCO 60%.

Arterial oxygen saturation was 96% at rest and 92% on walking 100 metres.

a) What is the most likely diagnosis?
b) How would you confirm your diagnosis?

31 A The diagram below indicates the relationship of affected and unaffected members of a family with a rare enzyme defect.

■ Affected   □ Unaffected

a) How is the condition inherited?

31 B a) In what Mendelian manner is this genetic trait transmitted?

b) Assuming penetrance is complete and that none of the family marries another carrier or affected individual, what is the risk of patients A, B, and C being affected? What would you estimate the risk to their children is?

c) List 5 important conditions transmitted in this way.

32 A 44 year old woman returns from Sri Lanka, having resided there for 5 years. Four months prior to leaving she developed an acute attack of gastroenteritis which settled initially. She then developed persistent colicky abdominal pain associated with loose bulky-stool diarrhoea and weight loss. She was investigated in Sri Lanka without success and was treated with oral metronidazole for presumed giardiasis. More recently she developed generalized aches and pains.

On examination she was clinically anaemic and pigmented. Abdominal examination was normal. Neurologically there was evidence of a proximal myopathy; in addition ankle jerks were absent and there was loss of vibration sense distally.

Investigations:

Hb	10.5 g/dl
MCV	108 fl
MCHC	32 g/dl
WBC	11×10^9/l
Albumin	29 g/l
Alkaline phosphatase	265 iu/l
Calcium	2.1 mmol/l
Phosphate	0.7 mmol/l
Aspartate aminotransferase	15 iu/l
Faecal fat	25 mmol/l
Stools	negative for ova cysts and parasites.

a) What is the most likely diagnosis?
b) Give a differential diagnosis.
c) How would you treat this patient?

Question 33

33 A 70 year old man presented with dull aching in both calves after moderate exercise. The symptoms had started 9 months earlier. Symptoms developed after walking 300–400 yards and settled after 5 minutes' rest, and would settle immediately if he sat down and stooped forward. Often, in addition to pain, he developed bilateral numbness in his thighs. He had no sphincter disturbance. He had had low back pain for many years. He had been depressed since his wife died. He smoked 20 cigarettes a day and was followed by a chest clinic for chronic obstructive airways disease. Medication included paracetamol as required, lofepramine 70 mg daily and two puffs from a salbutamol inhaler q.d.s.

On examination there was no rash, lymphadenopathy, clubbing, cyanosis or anaemia. His chest was clear, the heart sounds were normal, and the abdomen soft with no abnormal masses palpable. On inspection there was loss of his lumbar lordosis and reduced flexion and extension of the lumbar spine. Neurological examination of the cranial nerves and the upper limbs was normal. In the lower limbs tone power and coordination were normal; the reflexes were symmetrical but reduced compared to the upper limbs. The plantar reflexes were flexor. Soft touch and pin prick sensation were reduced from below the groin to just above the knees laterally. Proprioception and vibration sense were normal. The femoral, popliteal, posterior tibial and dorsalis anterior arterial pulses were present both at rest and after excercise.

Investigations:

Hb	14 g/dl
WBC	$7.5 \times 10^9/l$
Platelets	$455 \times 10^9/l$
Sodium	141 mmol/l
Potassium	3.9 mmol/l
Urea	7 mmol/l
Albumin	40 g/l
Calcium	2.3 mmol/l
Bilirubin	8 μmol/l
Aspartate transaminase	29 iu/l
Alkaline phosphatase	90 iu/l
IgG	15.5 g/l
IgA	2.2 g/l
IgM	3.0 g/l
Protein electrophoresis	normal
Bence-Jones protein	negative
CXR	consistent with mild obstructive airways disease
Lumbar spine X-ray	lumbar spondylosis with marked osteophyte formation

a) What is the most likely diagnosis?

b) What investigation would you do next to confirm this?

34 This M-mode echocardiogram is taken across the mid left ventricle. A is the left ventricular cavity and B is the interventricular septum.

a) What is abnormal about space A?

b) What is abnormal about space C?

c) Give two clinical signs that may be associated with space C.

1 cm marker

35 A 32 year old air-hostess presented with a 1-week history of fever and a migratory polyarthritis. For the last 2 days her left ankle and both knees had been painful and swollen but the other joints had settled. She had also developed tenosynovitis affecting the dorsum of her left hand. She was taking the oral contraceptive pill only. On direct questioning she had no other cardiorespiratory, abdominal, genitourinary or neurological symptoms.

On examination she had a hot swollen left ankle and left knee. Her right knee was tender only. In addition she had several vesicopustular lesions on her trunk, arms and lower legs.

Investigations:

Hb	14.5 g/dl
WBC	$12 \times 10^9/l$
Urea and electrolytes	normal
Rheumatoid factor	negative
Antinuclear factor	negative
Synovial aspiration	turbid fluid containing 35 000 neutrophils/ml
Blood cultures	negative
Synovial fluid	negative

a) What is the diagnosis?

b) How would you confirm your diagnosis?

36 A 25 year old woman becomes profoundly unwell with diarrhoea and is brought to casualty.

On examination she is drowsy, neck stiffness is absent and no focal neurological signs are detected. Temperature 39°C, heart rate 110, blood pressure 70/20 mmHg. Marked bilateral conjunctivitis, and a widespread macular rash are apparent.

Investigations:

Hb	14.5 g/dl
WBC	$14 \times 10^9/l$
Platelets	$100 \times 10^9/l$
Urea	10 mmol/l
Creatinine	158 µmol/l
Potassium	5 mmol/l
Creatinine phosphokinase	400 u/l

a) What is the likely diagnosis?

b) How would you confirm your diagnosis?

c) How would you treat the patient?

37A A 45 year old woman undergoing treatment for depression was admitted to hospital. She was drowsy and had a marked tremor. ECG on admission showed flat T-waves.

Investigations:

Sodium	148 mmol/l
Potassium	4 mmol/l
Urea	14 mmol/l
T4	59 nmol/l
TSH	12 mU/l

a) What is the likely diagnosis?

37B a) What is the likely cause of this patient's coma?
b) Explain the abnormal investigations.

Sodium	114 mmol/l
Potassium	4.1 mmol/l
Urea	2.8 mmol/l
Creatinine	106 µmol/l
Aspartate aminotransferase	138 iu/l
Hb	11 g/dl
MCV	104 fl
WBC	5×10^9/l
Platelets	42×10^9/l
Cholesterol	6.4 mmol/l
Triglyceride	3.4 mmol/l

38 A 20 year old girl presented to outpatients complaining of recurrent generalized itching and shortness of breath. In recent months she had had 3 episodes of pleurisy and mild shortness of breath on exertion. Her friends had commented to her that her holiday tan had lasted well into the winter. In the past she had experienced mild Raynaud's phenomenon which had required no treatment. She worked in an office and was not exposed to industrial dusts or chemicals. She took no regular medication and was a non-smoker. Her two maternal aunts had rheumatoid arthritis.

Examination revealed a fit-looking young woman who was well tanned. The skin on her forearms and fingers was boggy and oedematous but there was no desquamation. She had no lymphadenopathy, cyanosis, anaemia, clubbing or clinical jaundice. Her pulse was 80 regular, BP 150/90 mmHg, the jugular venous pressure was visible 1 cm above the angle of Louis. Her heart sounds were normal and there were several fine bilateral crackles heard at both lung bases.

Investigations:

Hb	13 g/dl
ESR	20 mm in the first hour
CRP	10 mg/l
Urea	4.6 mmol/l
Creatinine	145 μmol/l
Rheumatoid factor	negative
Antinuclear antibody	1/80 homogeneous
Complement profile	normal
Serum angiotensin-converting enzyme	normal
Chest X-ray	bilateral fine linear shadowing/atelectasis
Ventilation/perfusion scan	normal
Lung function tests	
FEV1	2.0 l
VC	2.4 l
PEFR	5.5 l/s
TLC	3.0 l
TLCO	80% predicted (80%)
VA	1.8 l (70%)
KCO	90% predicted

a) What is the most likely diagnosis?
b) What complications have occurred?

39 A 35 year old woman was seen in casualty with a perianal abscess. On direct questioning she had had a number of episodes of diarrhoea in the past 2–3 years which had been treated by her doctor with loperamide and courses of antibiotics (including metronidazole). At the age of 9 months she had had pneumonia, which was followed throughout her childhood by numerous chest infections and occasional crops of boils. She thought that her family was generally subject to boils and attributed this to a poor diet, since her father had been unemployed. Her only other complaint was 'rheumatics' – she had a long history of joint pains and occasional joint swellings, affecting mostly the large peripheral joints and the wrists, but not the small joints in her hands or feet. Her only medication was Nuseals-aspirin as required for her joint symptoms.

Examination showed a cheerful but thin lady with no clubbing, anaemia or lymphadenopathy. Examination of her joints revealed mild crepitus in both knees and limited rotation and extension of both hips. Her neck and lumbar spine were normal for her age. The cardiovascular system and CNS were normal. Her spleen was just palpable. Rectal examination confirmed a perianal abscess.

Investigations:

Hb	12 g/dl
WBC	$4.0 \times 10^9/l$ – 55% neutrophils, 40% lymphocytes
Platelets	$200 \times 10^9/l$
ESR	15 mm in the first hour
Sodium	135 mmol/l
Potassium	4.0 mmol/l
Urea	5.0 mmol/l
Creatinine	130 µmol/l
Albumin	43 g/l
Total protein	60 g/l
Aspartate amino-transferase	20 iu/l
Alkaline phosphatase	90 iu/l
Bilirubin	6 µmol/l
Rheumatoid factor and ANA	negative
Cultures of blood and stool	negative
Culture of the abscess	S. faecalis
Chest X-ray	normal
X-rays of knees and hips	early osteoarthritis
Abdominal ultrasound	splenomegaly

a) What is the diagnosis?

b) What investigation would you request?

c) What treatments are of value?

40 A 27 year old woman presents with a 2-day history of bleeding gums. On examination there are subconjunctival haemorrhages and patches of purpura.

Investigations:

Hb	6.4 g/dl
WBC	32.5 × 10⁹/l
Platelets	32 × 10⁹/l
Prothrombin time	20 s
APPT	50 s
Thrombin time	38 s
Fibrinogen	0.5 g/l

Film: numerous hypergranular promyelocytes present.

a) What is the likely diagnosis?

b) How would you confirm this diagnosis?

41 **A** A 50 year old man complains of exertional dyspnoea. The following lung function results are obtained:

FEV 23%, VC 56%, FEV/VC 33 (40%), TLCO 69%, KCO 73%, VA 96%

a) Name 2 other useful pulmonary function tests.

b) What is the most probable diagnosis?

B The following lung function tests were obtained in a 55 year old woman who was treated 10 years ago for an adenocarcinoma of the right main bronchus. She has remained well since then and is a non-smoker.

FEV 49%, VC 52%, FEV/VC 83 (98%), DLCO 75%, KCO 150%, VA 50%

a) How was her lung tumour treated?

C A 65 year old man has a history of bony tuberculosis as a young man, resulting in gibbus deformity of the thoracic spine. He is admitted to hospital with increasing breathlessness and confusion. Admission blood gases were as follows:

pH 7.41, pCO$_2$ 8.9 kPa, pO$_2$ 6.1 kPa, Bicarbonate 42 mmol/l

a) What is his respiratory problem?

b) What is the acid–base disturbance?

42 A 16 year old boy is brought into A&E with a short history of severe headache and vomiting. He has a widespread maculopapular rash all over his body, and is very drowsy. He is staying with relatives away from home, and his parents are abroad. His uncle thinks that he may have been admitted to hospital on two previous occasions with similar problems, but does not know any details. The patient is too unwell to give a coherent history.

a) What other signs should be sought?

b) What initial investigations are required? How would the results influence your management? What is the probable diagnosis?

c) What therapy would you initiate in this patient? What complications may occur in this condition?

d) What other tests are required at a later date? What underlying problem needs to be considered in this patient?

43 A 32 year old man presents with uncomfortable 'gritty' eyes, and painful knees – particularly on weight-bearing. He has just returned from a business trip to Bangkok.

a) What other questions would you ask when taking an initial history from this man?

b) What is the probable diagnosis? What important differential should be considered?

c) What other signs should be sought?

d) What other factors predispose to this condition?

44 A 39 year old publican presents with a 6-month history of headache and malaise. He smokes 20 cigarettes a day, drinks regularly throughout the day and is on a thiazide diuretic for the treatment of mild hypertension. On examination he is plethoric and hypertensive, blood pressure 190/115 mmHg. He has 3 cm hepatomegaly and 4 cm splenomegaly.

Investigations:

Hb	20.9 g/dl
WBC	$14.9 \times 10^9/l$
Platelets	$517 \times 10^9/l$
Sodium	143 mmol/l
Potassium	4 mmol/l
Urea	4.3 mmol/l
Bilirubin	24 µmol/l
Aspartate transaminase	63 iu/l
Alkaline phosphatase	163 iu/l
Uric acid	0.6 mmol/l
PO_2	12.8 kPa
pCO_2	5.3 kPa
PH	7.42

a) What is the likely diagnosis?

b) What further investigations are appropriate?

45 This 13 year old underwent cardiac catheterization. Her parents had noticed that she was becoming increasingly breathless and blue.

	SAT O$_2$(%)	PRESS (mmHg)
RA	74	26 Mean
RV	76	110/5–10
PA	76	110/30
LV	92	105/0–10
Aorta	99	120/75

a) What waveform do you expect in the right atrial pressure trace and why?

b) Is the pulmonary valve functioning normally?

c) Describe any changes that you would expect between the vascular markings on the chest X-rays at 1 year and now.

46 A 48 year old woman was admitted to hospital with a 3-week history of intermittent fever, profound weakness, severe myalgia and arthralgia. The illness had begun with influenza-like symptoms and a mild sore throat. The fever was worse in the evening and generally lasted less than 12 hours. Oral amoxycillin and then tetracycline had been prescribed without effect. She denied respiratory or cardiovascular symptoms, had no abdominal pain, diarrhoea, urinary frequency, dysuria or urgency, headache, neck stiffness or photophobia. There was no significant past medical history. There was no history of travel abroad. Her grandmother had had rheumatoid arthritis. She took no medication regularly, smoked 10 cigarettes per day and drank little alcohol.

Temperature 40°C, pulse 105 regular, BP 110/70 mmHg, respiratory rate 20/min. There was no rash, petechiae or lymphadenopathy. There were white patches in her mouth which on culture proved to be *candida albicans*. There was no anaemia, cyanosis or jaundice; she had no clubbing or oedema. Examination of the chest and cardiovascular system revealed only a soft pansytolic murmur best heard at the apex. Her breasts and thyroid were normal. Palpation of the abdomen revealed splenomegaly. Her right knee had a warm effusion and both wrists were painful. Neurological examination was normal. Three days after admission she developed a fine non-prusitic erythematous macular rash on her arms and neck; the rash changed its distribution on the arms and upper trunk each day and exhibited Koebner's phenomenon. The patient was started on indomethacin 25 mg t.d.s. with rapid resolution of the fever and pains.

Investigations:
Haematology:
Hb 10.5 g/dl, MCV 82 fl, WBC 12 × 10⁹/l – 85% neutrophils, Platelets 250 × 10⁹/l, ESR 120 mm in the first hour
Biochemistry:
Sodium 138 mmol/l, Potassium 4.0 mmol/l, Bicarbonate 25 mmol/l, Urea 5.0 mmol/l, Bilirubin 12.0 μmol/l, Aspartate transaminase 30 iu/l, Alkaline phosphatase 60 iu/l, Total protein 75 g/l, Albumin 38 g/l, CRP 65 mg/l, Creatinine kinase 35 iu/l, Glucose 4 mmol/l

Other investigations:
ANA and Rheumatoid factor negative.
VDRL negative, ASOT negative, Heterophile antibodies negative, CMV antibodies not detected
Synovial fluid – thin and contained high numbers of neutrophils
Throat culture – candida only. Cultures of blood, urine, stool and synovial fluid were negative
Urine dipstick negative
Chest X-ray normal
X-rays of the knees and wrists normal apart from soft tissue swelling of the right knee.
ECG and echocardiogram normal

X-rays of the knees and wrists normal apart from soft tissue swelling of the right knee.
ECG and echocardiogram normal
a) What is the most likely diagnosis?
b) What further investigations would you request?

47 You are asked to see a 69 year old Hepatitis B-positive Asian man on the ward who has been receiving chemotherapy for peritoneal tuberculosis. He has become increasingly weak and his urine output has decreased dramatically over the previous week. He has a temperature of 38.4°C, and is complaining of pains in his wrists and elbows. His serum creatinine is 456 μmol/l, urea 23.1 mmol/l and potassium 2.4 mmol/l. Urinalysis shows + RBC, ++WBC, and + protein.
a) What further information should be obtained in the history?
b) What is the likely diagnosis? Why?
c) What other blood tests are required?
d) What other investigations are needed, and what findings would you expect?
e) What therapy is needed? Assuming that the patient requires renal replacement therapy acutely, what factors in the history may be relevant?

48 This patient has had recurrent syncope and heart failure.

12.5 mm/sec; 0.5 cm/mV

a) What is demonstrated?
b) If there is nothing different on the 24-hour tape what difference in prognosis would be achieved by abolishing the arrhythmia pharmacologically?

49 A 57 year old obese man is referred to outpatients with a history of visual disturbance. On two occasions he described transient loss of vision in the left eye. This came on over a few seconds, gradually obscuring all vision in that eye. After 3 or 4 minutes the vision cleared completely. On one occasion during an attack he was at his desk writing with his right hand, and noticed that his handwriting seemed to deteriorate, and he had difficulty holding his pen.

a) What is the likely diagnosis?

b) What other facts would you try to elicit in the history?

c) What physical signs should be sought?

d) How would you manage this patient?

e) What is the commonest cause of death in these patients?

50 A 37 year old trout farmer presents with a 7-day history of fever, myalgias, nausea and severe frontal headache. He has experienced occasional colicky abdominal pain and vomited once. On two occasions he has noticed haematuria. One month previously he returned from his honeymoon in France but has not otherwise travelled abroad. At the age of 6 he suffered an episode of infectious hepatitis and there is a family history of diabetes mellitus. He drinks 5 pints of beer most evenings but does not smoke. He takes paracetamol occasionally for long-standing lower back pain.

On examination he is pyrexial 38.5°C and icteric. Bilateral subconjunctival haemorrhages and a purpuric rash over both calves are noted. There is no asterixis and he is alert. He has marked photophobia but no neck stiffness. In the abdomen he has smooth 4 cm hepatomegaly.

Investigations:

Hb	11.3 g/dl
WBC	15.9 × 10⁹/l – 90% neutrophils
Platelets	470 × 10⁹/l
Sodium	132 mmol/l
Potassium	4.5 mmol/l
Urea	27.8 mmol/l
Creatinine	305 µmol/l
Bilirubin	76 µmol/l
Aspartate amino-transferase	78 iu/l
Alkaline phosphatase	642 iu/l
PT	13 s
PTTK	32 s
Urine dipstick	protein++, blood++
Urine microscopy	occasional white cells, occasional red cells, no casts

a) What is the likely diagnosis?

b) How would you confirm your diagnosis?

c) What treatment would you recommend?

51 A 54 year old man presents with a 4-hour history of severe, retrosternal chest pain and increasing shortness of breath. The pain started suddenly whilst eating, is constant in nature and radiates to the neck and interscapular region. In 1980 he was found to be hypertensive and is currently taking nifedipine slow release 20 mg b.d. There is no other significant past medical history and no previous history of chest tightness. He smokes 20 cigarettes a day and drinks up to 6 pints of beer a day.

On examination he is distressed and clammy. Pulse 110 and regular, blood pressure 85/50 supine, JVP not elevated, heart sounds normal. All peripheral pulses are present and symmetrical. The left lung base is dull to percussion and breath sounds are decreased. Abdominal and neurological examination is normal. ECG shows sinus tachycardia and T-wave inversion in lead III. Chest X-ray shows a small left pleural effusion.

a) What is the diagnosis? Give a differential diagnosis.

b) How would you confirm your diagnosis?

52 A 45 year old mentally subnormal woman presents in casualty with a broken arm after repeated falls. She has had epilepsy since childhood. Her last witnessed fit was 2 weeks ago; before this she had been fit-free for 2 years. Pulmonary tuberculosis had been diagnosed 6 months previously. Her medication consisted of phenytoin 400 mg, primidone 200 mg and Rifinah (combined rifampicin and isoniazid) 2 tablets daily.

Examination confirmed the fracture. In addition she had mild nystagmus and ataxia. Otherwise physical examination was normal.

Investigations:

Hb	11 g/l
MCV	105 fl
WBC	8×10^9/l – normal differential
Platelets	400×10^9/l
Sodium	136 mmol/l
Potassium	4.0 mmol/l
Urea	5 mmol/l
Albumin	40 g/l
Calcium	2.1 mmol/l
Phosphate	1.0 mmol/l
Bilirubin	6 μmol/l
Aspartate transaminase	28 iu/l
Alkaline phosphatase	180 iu/l

a) What is the diagnosis?

b) What investigations would you perform?

53 A A 29 year old woman presents with progressive breathlessness on exertion of 6 months' duration. Pulmonary function tests are performed:

FEV 90%, VC 92%, FEV/VC 96%, DLCO 59%, KCO 65%, VA 91%

On exercise, arterial saturation measured by oximetry fell from 94% to 86% at 55% of predicted maximum workload.

a) Give 2 possible diagnoses.
b) Suggest 2 other relevant investigations.

B A 58 year old man with rheumatoid arthritis complains of progressive breathlessness on exertion. On examination he is centrally cyanosed with fine crackles at both lung bases. Lung function results are as follows:

FEV 59%, VC 52%, FEV/VC 113%, TLC 80%, RV 77%, DLCO 23%, KCO 42%, VA 61%

a) What is the most likely diagnosis?
b) Name 2 useful further investigations.

54 A 24 year old man is brought into casualty in a semiconscious state after a football match on a Saturday afternoon. He smells strongly of drink.

a) What signs may be observed?
b) It seem likely that the patient is suffering from alcohol poisoning. What other possibilities must be considered?
c) What complications may ensue?
d) How would you treat this patient?

55 A 29 year old woman presents to the clinic with a short history of headaches, which are worse in the morning, and double vision. On examination, the patient weighs 102 kg, there is papilloedema, and a partial right VI nerve palsy, but no other abnormal neurological signs.

a) What is the most likely diagnosis? Why? What other important possibility must be excluded?
b) What urgent investigation is required?
c) What is the main risk in this condition?
d) What is the treatment?

56 This patient is in casualty 2 hours after the onset of chest pain.

a) Predict the appearance of the coronary arteriogram.

b) What feature suggests that streptokinase has been given?

c) What would be the significance of a period of atrioventricular nodal dissociation?

d) What would you expect if the ECG has not changed in 1 year's time?

Limb leads

Chest leads   19 mm/sec; 0.75 cm/mV

57 This data was acquired from cardiac catheterization of a 26
year old man with episodic dizziness.

	SAT O$_2$(%)	Press (mmHg)
RA	73	Mean 5
		A-wave 7
RV	75	97/0–10
PA	74	24/14
LV	96	130/0–10
Femoral artery	92	185/60

a) What is the most likely cause for the systemic desaturation?
b) What is the valve lesion?
c) Echocardiography shows a thick ventricular wall. What other
abnormality do you suspect?
d) Give 3 possible causes for the dizzy spells.

58 A 34 year old man presents with a 1-week history of pain in the left eye, associated with blurred vision. One year before, he had noticed that his ability to play tennis had been transiently impaired by apparent weakness of his right foot, but he had not sought medical advice as the symptoms had resolved after about a month. He had, however, been treated by his GP for acute labyrinthitis about 3 months before developing his current problem.

a) What is the likely diagnosis?

b) What signs might be elicited on examination of the eyes?

c) How would you interpret the patient's history prior to this acute presentation?

d) What investigations are required?

e) What is the prognosis of the ocular lesion? What will be the appearance of the optic disc 6 months later?

59 An 8 year old boy is admitted following a grand mal convulsion. Routine blood investigations:

Glucose	4 mmol/l
Calcium	1.7 mmol/l
Albumin	39 g/l
Phosphate	1.9 mmol/l
Alkaline phosphatase	190 iu/l
Urea	4 mmol/l
Creatinine	75 μmol/l
Hb	11 g/dl

a) What is the cause of his convulsion?

b) Give a differential diagnosis and describe how you would investigate further.

60 A 60 year old woman with hypertension presented to her GP complaining of increasing fatigue and chest pains for the last 3 months. The chest pains were intermittent, sharp in nature and localized over the precordium. Occasionally she was woken at night by chest pain, which was relieved by sitting forwards. Recently she had developed aching joints. Her medication was atenolol 100 mg o.d., bendrofluazide 2.5 mg b.d., hydrallazine 50 mg q.d.s. On examination her BP was well controlled at 130/80 mmHg, her heart sounds were normal and there were no added sounds. She had a mild rash over both cheeks and the back of her hands which she attributed to chemicals she used in the garden.

Investigations:

Hb	12 g/dl
WBC	$3.0 \times 10^9/l$
Platelets	$150 \times 10^9/l$
ESR	50 mm in the first hour
Rheumatoid factor	negative
ANA	1/160 homogeneous
Immunoglobulins	normal
CXR	small bilateral pleural effusions and a large heart
ECG	sinus rhythm, normal QRS complexes but of low voltage, small or inverted T-waves in most leads

a) What is the most likely diagnosis?
b) What treatment would you advise?

61 This is data acquired at cardiac catheterization of a 32 year old woman with dyspnoea.

	Sat O_2(%)	Press (mmHg)
RA	73	Mean 6 A-wave 10
RV	74	60/0–10
PA	73	Mean 50
PACW		Mean 26 A-Wave 32 End diastole 19
LV	98	120/0–10
Aorta	99	120/75

a) What is the primary lesion demonstrated?
b) Explain the high A-wave pressure in the right atrial measurement.
c) What may be palpated at the precordium?
d) What is the underlying cardiac rhythm?

62 A 40 year old man was admitted for investigation of an abnormal chest X-ray which showed persistent linear shadowing and a solitary nodular shadow in the left lower lobe. He had a dry cough, occasional fever and had lost 4 kg in weight over a 3-month period. He smoked 20 cigarettes per day and drank 2–3 pints of beer per day. He worked in the construction industry installing roofs. Recently he had been exposed to considerable amounts of tile dust and in the past he had been exposed to asbestos. One year before he had returned from a holiday pot-holing in France and developed an acute illness characterized by flitting arthralgia, a cough, left-sided chest pain, erythema nodosum, fever and malaise. A chest X-ray was reported as showing pneumonia and he received a course of penicillin and then oxytetracyclin. However his symptoms settled slowly and he was discharged home after 3 weeks.

On examination his temperature was 37.5°C, pulse 74 regular and BP 110/70 mmHg. There was no palpable lymphadenopathy, cyanosis, anaemia, jaundice or clubbing. Examination of the chest revealed a normal heart and an area of dullness with decreased breath sounds at the left lung base. Abdominal and CNS examination were normal.

Investigations:

Hb	14 g/dl
WBC	11.8 × 10^9/l – neutrophils 85%
Platelets	400 × 10^9/l
Urea and electrolytes	normal
Glucose	5.3 mmol/l
Aspartate amino-transferase	28 iu/l
Alkaline phosphatase	130 iu/l
Bilirubin	6.0 μmol/l
Total protein	70 g/l
Albumin	30 g/l
Serum angiotensin-converting enzyme	normal
Tuberculin test	negative
Repeated blood cultures	negative
Lung function tests	within normal limits
ECG	normal

Chest X-ray: A single, well-defined, non-calcified nodule with several linear shadows in the left lower lung field with marked pleural thickening. There was no hilar lymph node enlargement Bronchoscopy – no endobronchial masses. Washings: no malignant cells, macrophages+; culture negative for bacteria and tuberculosis.

An ultrasound-guided needle biopsy of the pleura and lung tissue was obtained. Microscopic examination of the material revealed no malignant cells and no acid-fast bacteria. There were several necrotizing granulomas with multinucleated giant cells and marked fibrosis.

a) What is the most likely diagnosis?
b) List 3 other important differential diagnoses.
c) Suggest 2 investigations.

63 A 26 year old woman attends outpatients with a 2-month history of left hip pain – worse on weight-bearing and on exertion. Some relief is obtained from Ibuprofen. She has a complex previous medical history: 18 months previously she underwent a trans-sphenoidal hypophysectomy for a benign pituitary lesion which has resulted in pituitary failure. She had been on thyroid replacement therapy with 150 μg T_4 for two years, and oestrogen therapy for 9 months. Perioperatively she had received 4 mg q.d.s. of dexamethasone for 3 weeks, and had been taking 2 mg b.d. for the last 12 months. Her weight was 102 kg; height 5ft 1 inch.

a) What is the most likely explanation for her hip pain? What other joints may be affected in this condition?
b) What investigations would you perform?
c) Was her endocrine replacement therapy entirely appropriate? Why might this be relevant?

64A A 55 year old man presents with a 12-hour history of severe abdominal pain and vomiting. He had been recently commenced on a thiazide diuretic for high blood pressure. On examination he was unwell, sweaty and tachycardic, with a blood pressure of 115/85 mmHg. His abdomen was diffusely tender and bowel sounds were absent.

Investigations:

Hb	13 g/dl
WBC	14 × 10^9/l
Platelets	245 × 10^9/l
Sodium	143 mmol/l
Potassium	3.9 mmol/l
Urea	9 mmol/l
Albumin	27 g/l
Calcium	1.9 mmol/l
Phosphate	0.8 mmol/l
Bilirubin	25 μmol/l
Aspartate transaminase	40 iu/l
Glucose	13 mmol/l
pO_2	8.8 kPa
pCO_2	4.0 kPa

a) What is the likely diagnosis and how would you confirm your diagnosis?
b) Suggest a possible cause in this case.

64B A 49 year old smoker is admitted to casualty having had a seizure at work. His colleagues describe a typical grand mal fit. The patient gives a further history of increasingly frequent severe headaches in recent months, and also difficulty in concentrating at work. His wife had noticed that he had been taking a good deal of time off, and seemed unusually cheerful and impulsive.
a) What is the probable diagnosis?
b) Which features in the history are important?
c) What investigations would you perform?

65 A 35 year old woman is admitted confused, pyrexial and vomiting. Her flat-mate reports that she has been unwell for the last three months and has lost weight. Three days previously she was bed bound with a severe cold. Her brother who was called urgently by the flat-mate, collapsed in casualty, and was found to be hypoglycaemic. He responded to intravenous dextrose, it transpired that he missed his evening meal in his rush to visit his sister. He has been insulin dependent for 5 years.

On examination the sister is disorientated in time and place, temperature 39°C, pulse 110 irregularly irregular with a blood pressure of 100/60. There is no neck stiffness and no focal neurological signs. The duty SHO has performed a lumbar puncture.

Investigations:

Hb	14 g/dl
WBC	9×10^9/l – 70% neutrophils
Sodium	140 mmol/l
Potassium	4 mmol/l
Urea	13 mmol/l
Albumin	35 g/l
Calcium	2.6 mmol/l
Phosphate	1.2 mmol/l
Glucose	5.2 mmol/l
CSF	Opening pressure 9 cm water
	Protein 0.6 g/l
	Glucose 4 mmol/l
	Cell count 3 lymphocytes/mm3

a) What is the likely diagnosis?
b) How would you treat the patient?

66 A 28 year old woman is admitted with a right deep vein thrombosis. Three years ago a left deep vein thrombosis was diagnosed, she was anticoagulated for 6 months and the oral contraceptive pill was stopped. The past medical history is otherwise unremarkable apart from 2 spontaneous mid-trimester abortions.

Investigations:

Hb	13 g/dl
WBC	$6 \times 10^9/l$
Platelets	$90 \times 10^9/l$
Urea and electrolytes	normal
Admission clotting profile	
PT	12 s
APTT	65 s
Complement levels	normal
ANF	negative

Antibodies to extractable nuclear antigens not detected.

a) What is the likely diagnosis?

b) What are the other recognized associations?

c) What further tests would you ask for to confirm your diagnosis?

67A A 35 year old woman is admitted to casualty with status epilepticus. The convulsion is terminated with diazepam. On recovering consciousness she gives a history of severe abdominal pain and vomiting and admits to having had 2 previous fits. She has noted progressive weakness in her right arm and is unable to grip a tennis racquet properly. On examination she looks well, is apyrexial with a regular pulse and blood pressure. There are no localizing signs in the abdomen. Neurologically there is a right radial nerve palsy – the rest of the examination is unremarkable.

Investigations:

Sodium	123 mmol/l
Potassium	4.0 mmol/l
Urea	4 mmol/l
Bilirubin	35 µmol/l
Aspartate transaminase	42 iu/l

a) Suggest a unifying diagnosis.

b) How would you confirm this diagnosis?

67B A 3 week old infant is seen with vomiting, diarrhoea and failure to thrive. On examination there is hepatomegaly and early cataracts are noted.

Blood glucose   1.9 mmol/l

a) What is the likely diagnosis?
b) What are the other recognized complications?
c) How would you confirm your diagnosis?
d) What treatment would you advocate?

68 A 65 year old woman was referred to outpatients with a 3-month history of progressive vertigo which was worse when she turned her head to the left. For two months she had had intermittent tinnitus and dull occipital headaches. General enquiry revealed that she had lost 4 kg of weight over 9 months, felt depressed and had lost her appetite. There was no relevant respiratory or cardiovascular history, no recent change in bowel habit and no genitourinary symptoms. She took bendrofluazide 2.5 mg daily and atenolol 50 mg daily for hypertension. In the past she had had an appendicectomy and a benign lump removed from her right breast. She was a lifelong non-smoker and consumed little alcohol.

Examination: weight 65 kg, temperature 37°C. There was no clubbing, cyanosis, jaundice or lymphadenopathy. There were no thyroid or breast masses. Pulse 60 regular, blood pressure 150/70 mmHg, heart and lungs normal. Examination of the abdomen revealed an appendicetomy scar only. She was well-orientated but had mild dysarthria and memory impairment. On walking she was clumsy and needed help to climb on to the couch; when walking in a straight line she tended to veer to the right. On right lateral gaze she had right beat nystagmus and several beats of rotatory nystagmus looking to the left. She had bilateral sensorineural deafness. Otherwise examination of the cranial nerves was normal. She had normal power and tone in all limbs. Both deep and superficial reflexes were symmetrical and normal. Coordination in her upper limbs was normal; there was no tremor and no dysdiadochokinesis. Sensation was normal.

Investigations:

Haematology
Hb 11 g/dl, MCV 84 fl, WBC 9.0 × 10^9/l, Platelets 400 × 10^9/l, ESR 35 mm in the first hour.

Biochemistry
Sodium 140 mmol/l, Potassium 3.3 mmol/l, Urea 5.0 mmol/l, Creatinine 90 μmol/l, Bilirubin 6.0 μmol/l, Aspartate aminotransferase 15 iu/l, Alkaline phosphatase 60 iu/l, Total protein 76 g/l, Albumin 41 g/l, Calcium 2.5 mmol/l, Phosphate 1.23 mmol/l, Creatinine kinase 35 iu/l, Glucose 6.0 mmol/l.

Other investigations
T4 80 nmol/l, ANA and rheumatoid factor negative. Syphilis
serology negative.
Urine dipstick – negative protein. No Bence-Jones proteins.
Lumbar puncture: CSF Glu 4.0 mmol/l, Protein 1.0 g/l,
WBC 20 mm³, no fungi or microorganisms seen.
Chest X-ray, calcification and pleural thickening in both lung
apices. Abdominal X-ray normal.
CT-head scan – cortical and cerebellar atrophy, no focal lesions
seen.
Abdominal ultrasound – minimal ascites, normal sized liver,
kidneys and spleen with normal architecture; no
lymphadenopathy; the right ovary contained several cysts
containing some calcification; the left ovary was not seen.
a) What is the most likely diagnosis?
b) What investigation would you perform next?

69 **A** A 10 year old boy complains of orthopnoea. Pulmonary
function tests reveal the following:
FEV1 68%, VC 70% erect, 37% supine
a) What abnormality is suggested by these results?
b) Give 2 possible underlying causes.

B A 25 year old woman presents with acute renal failure.
Diffuse interstitial shadowing is noted on CXR and she has
marked arterial hypoxaemia. Pulmonary function tests were as
follows:
FEV 75%, VC 67%, FEV/VC 114%, DLCO 173%, KCO 275%, VA
62%
a) What is the abnormality and what pathological process is
occurring?
b) Give 2 possible causes in this patient.

C A 53 year old man complains of difficulty in breathing, worse
in the morning and sometimes waking him at night. Lung
function tests are shown below:
FEV 57%, VC 93%, FEV/VC 63%, TLCO 116%, KCO 145%, VA
80%. Spirometry post-bronchodilator: FEV 92%, VC 101%, FEV/
VC 72 (93%)
a) What is the diagnosis?

70 A 65 year old man was seen in outpatients with a 3-month history of malaise, headache, myalgia, scalp tenderness, fever and weight loss. On examination vision was normal, both carotid arteries were tender to palpation. Routine blood investigations were normal but the ESR was elevated at 100 mm in the first hour. A clinical diagnosis of giant-cell arteritis was made and he was treated with 60 mg of prednisolone a day. Two months later he was still on 60 mg of prednisolone a day and his symptoms had not improved.

Investigations:

Hb	9.8 g/dl
MCV	82 fl
WBC	9 × 10⁹/l
Platelets	260 × 10⁹/l
ESR	123 mm in the first hour
Sodium	140 mmol/l
Potassium	4 mmol/l
Urea	3.7 mmol/l
Albumin	37 g/l
Bilirubin	23 iu/l
Aspartate aminotransferase	26 iu/l
Urine dipstick	protein++, blood +++

a) Do you agree with the initial diagnosis?

b) What diagnosis would you consider?

71 A 30 year old man presented with an acute history of blanching, coolness and parasthesiae affecting his entire left foot. For the last year he had had an intermittent ache in his left calf, worse during jogging. He had stopped working as a contract plumber 2 years before, after developing severe work-related Raynaud's phenomenon in his right hand which had caused him to lose the tip of his right second digit after a minor abrasion.

His general health was good and he was able to jog regularly, although he had given up squash because his right arm became painful during the game. His father had hypertension. There was no history of diabetes mellitus, rheumatic fever, hypertension, hepatitis, polio or trauma to his leg. He took no regular medication, smoked 15 cigarettes a day and drank little alcohol.

On examination he was not clubbed, there were no xanthomata, and no lymphadenopathy was found. The lungs and heart were normal, pulse 70 regular, BP 130/70 mmHg. He had no bruits. Palpation of the abdomen was normal. The carotid, brachial, femoral and popliteal pulses were equal and easily palpated (graded ++). His right radial and ulnar arteries were impalpable, those on the left were graded +. The posterior tibial and dorsalis pedis were present on the right, graded ++, and only just palpable on the left side. Neurological examination was normal apart from reduced pin-prick and soft touch sensation in his left toes.

Investigations:
Haematology
Hb 14 g/dl, WBC 6 × 10⁹/l, Platelets 500 × 10⁹/l, ESR 40 mm in the first hour.
Prothrombin time 8.0 s, control 10.5 s. APTT 30 s, control 25 s.
Biochemistry
Sodium 138 mmol/l, Potassium 4.0 mmol/l, Urea 5.0 mmol/l, Calcium 2.4 mmol/l, Total protein 75 g/l, Albumin 45 g/l, Bilirubin 4.0 μmol/l, Aspartate transaminase 30 iu/l, Alkaline phosphatase 130 iu/l, Creatinine kinase 35 iu/l, Amylase 20 iu/l, CRP 2 mg/l.
Other investigations:
Plasma cholesterol 4 mmol/l, Triglyceride 1.2 mmol/l
ANA negative, Latex negative
Urine NAD
CXR and AXR NAD. X-rays of the neck, thoracic outlet and lumbar spine were normal.
ECG normal. 2-D echocardiogram – normal chamber size, normal valves, no dyskinetic segments.
Digital subtraction angiography of the abdominal aorta and peripheral arteries: normal apart from slight irregularity of the left proximal popliteal artery followed by an abrupt occlusion.

There were several collateral vessels reconstituting the left tibioperoneal trunk, some of which were also blocked.
a) What is the likely diagnosis?
b) How would you treat this man?
c) What further investigations would you arrange?

72 This patient has been admitted to the ITU with progressive deterioration after an influenza-like illness. Swan–Ganz and radial artery cannulae are in place.

	Sat O_2(%)	Press (mmHg)
SVC	48	
IVC	43	
mRA	47	Mean 22
RV	48	30/12
PA	47	33/16
PCWP		Mean 29
		V-wave 39
Radial artery	98	74/50

a) Why is the patient cyanosed?
b) Why is the superior vena cava blood so desaturated, and why is it less desaturated than the inferior vena cava blood?
c) What single measurement confers some grounds for hope of possible recovery?
d) Does the radial artery saturation surprise you? What is the explanation?

73 A 30 year old woman was admitted with an upper gastrointestinal tract haemorrhage. She had had mild upper abdominal pain for 1 year; otherwise she was well. She was on no regular medication. She was unmarried, worked as a journalist, smoked 20 cigarettes per day and on average drank 2 glasses of wine per week.

On examination she was well tanned but had pale mucous membranes. There were two spider naevi on her upper trunk but no palmar erythema, jaundice or lymphadenopathy. Examination of the heart and lungs was normal. On palpation of her abdomen her liver was one finger-breadth below the costal margin and the tip of her spleen could be felt. Neurological examination was normal.

Investigations:

Hb	12.5 g/dl
WBC	5.5 × 10⁹/l
Platelets	200 × 10⁹/l
MCV	88 fl
ESR	40 mm in the first hour
Sodium	135 mmol/l
Potassium	4 mmol/l
Urea	5 mmol/l
Albumin	35 g/l
IgG	16 g/l
IgM	9 g/l
IgA	2 g/l
Calcium	1.9 mmol/l
Phosphate	0.6 mmol/l
Glucose	5.0 mmol/l
Bilirubin	12 μmol/l
Aspartate transaminase	30 iu/l
Alkaline phosphatase	300 iu/l
γ-GT	80 iu/l
Prothrombin time	12 s
Chest X-ray	normal
Abdominal X-ray	normal
Urinalysis	normal

a) Give the most likely underlying diagnosis.

b) What further investigations would you request?

Question 74

74 An 87 year old man presents with a 3-year history of intermittent diarrhoea. He denies abdominal pain and his appetite has been unimpaired but he has lost 2 stones in weight over this period. He has obstructive airways disease and a 30-year history of grand mal epilepsy which is well controlled by phenytoin. Seven years previously he underwent emergency surgery for acute abdominal pain and peritonitis. He lives alone and has a poor diet, including 2 pints of Guinness every day.

On examination he is pale and cachectic. Abdominal examination is normal apart from the presence of a central scar.

Investigations:

Hb	8.4 g/dl
WBC	$4.3 \times 10^9/l$
Platelets	$90 \times 10^9/l$
MCV	125 fl
Sodium	137 mmol/l
Potassium	4 mmol/l
Urea	4 mmol/l
Serum folate	22 µg/l
B_{12}	80 ng/l
Schilling test	5% pre-intrinsic factor
	6% post-intrinsic factor

a) What is the likely cause of the anaemia?

b) What further investigations would you perform to confirm this?

75 A 55 year old man was referred with an 8-month history of tiredness and mild ankle oedema. Eight years ago he had had a small anterior myocardial infarction from which he had made an uneventful recovery; he had had prostatic cancer diagnosed 9 months ago and an anxiety state diagnosed 2 years before. His medication was fosfestrol 200 mg t.d.s. and atenolol 100 mg daily.

On examination his pulse was 55 regular, BP 120/60 mmHg, he has cold peripheries but was not cyanosed. There was no anaemia, jaundice or lymphadenopathy. The jugular venous pressure was visible on expiration. Palpation of the precordium and first and second heart sounds were normal. He had mild ankle oedema and several inspiratory crackles in both bases. Examination of his neck, abdomen and nervous system were otherwise normal.

Investigations:

Hb	12 g/dl
WBC	5.0 × 10⁹/l
Sodium	139 mmol/l
Potassium	4 mmol/l
Urea	4.0 mmol/l
Creatinine	70 µmol/l
Albumin	35 g/l
T4	180 nmol/l
TSH	1.0 mu/l
Urinalysis	normal
CXR	normal heart size and clear lung fields
ECG	sinus rhythm, with normal QRS and T-wave inversion in leads V4-6.

a) What is the explanation for this patient's clinical problems?

b) What 2 investigations would you request?

76 A 52 year woman is admitted to casualty feeling unwell. She has a severe headache, which came on suddenly while she was watching television, and has vomited once. She is apyrexial, but has some neck stiffness and is rather drowsy. Pulse 100 sinus rhythm, BP 150/95 mmHg. She has no other focal neurological signs, and fundoscopy was normal.

a) What are the two main differential diagnoses? Which is the more likely, and why?

b) What is the most important initial investigation that is required? How will the results help to distinguish between the two main differential diagnoses?

c) What other tests should be performed urgently?

d) What is the commonest cause of this problem?

e) How would you manage this patient?

Question 77

77 A 36 year old housewife was admitted with 3-month history of difficulty in walking. She complained that her legs felt stiff and weak but she was otherwise well and had no significant past medical history. Her periods had been irregular and heavy since the birth of her 18 month old son. She smoked 20 cigarettes a day and drank 2 pints of stout a night.
On examination she avoided eye contact but higher mental function was normal. Gait was spastic in nature, tone was symmetrically increased in both legs, power was decreased in a pyramidal fashion, reflexes were brisk with bilateral clonus and extensor plantars. No sensory abnormality could be detected, abdominal reflexes were absent. Neurological examination of the arms and cranial nerves was normal. General examination was unremarkable.

Investigations:

Hb	8.3 g/dl
MCV	72 fl
MCH	26 pg
MCHC	28 g/dl
WBC	$5 \times 10^9/l$
Platelets	$237 \times 10^9/l$
ESR	5 mm in the first hour
Sodium	138 mmol/l
Potassium	4 mmol/l
Urea	4 mmol/l
Albumin	40 g/l
Calcium	2.7 mmol/l
Aspartate amino-transferase	23 iu/l
Alkaline phosphatase	123 iu/l
Bilirubin	8 µmol/l
Chest X-ray	well-defined circular lesion overlying the left pulmonary artery
Thoracic spine X-ray	normal
Lung function tests	low DLCO and KCO (for Hb 8.3 g/dl)

a) Give a differential diagnosis. What is the most likely diagnosis?

b) What is the single most important investigation to perform? List 3 other investigations you would perform.

78A A 65 year old woman develops persistent diarrhoea. On examination she appears to have a migratory erythematous rash over her legs.

Investigations:

Hb	9 g/dl
WBC	11 × 10⁹/l
Platelets	230 × 10⁹/l
Glucose	10 mmol/l

a) Give a unifying diagnosis
b) How would you confirm your diagnosis?
c) How would you manage the patient?

78B A 35 year old male solicitor is referred by his GP. He was diagnosed as being hypertensive 1 year ago and despite drug treatment including β-blockers, calcium antagonists and an ACE inhibitor, his blood pressure remains elevated. He drinks 4 pints of beer per day and smokes 2 cigars every evening.

In the clinic, supine blood pressure is recorded as 210/110 mmHg. Fundi – grade III retinopathy. The rest of the examination is normal.

Investigations:

Sodium	148 mmol/l
Potassium	3.0 mmol/l
Bicarbonate	32 mmol/l
Urea	4 mmol/l
Glucose	4 mmol/l
Urine	negative protein

a) What is the likely diagnosis?
b) What further investigations are indicated?

79 The affected members in this family were below the 3rd
   centile in height and had a plasma phosphate consistently
   below 0.45 mmol/l; their alkaline phosphotase was between 150
   and 200 iu/l and their calcium was within the normal range.

■ Affected   □ Unaffected   ▨ Unknown

a) What is the diagnosis? How is the defect inherited?
b) What is the risk of A and B being affected?

80 A 26 year old woman presents to casualty after a series of grand mal fits. She had been well until the onset of fits 12 hours previously. On examination she has a temperature of 38°C, pulse 90, blood pressure 135/90 mmHg. Neurologically she is alert with a left VI nerve palsy and upper motor weakness of the right arm.

Investigations:

Hb	9.7 g/dl
WBC	$8.9 \times 10^9/l$
Platelets	$20 \times 10^9/l$
Blood film	red cell fragmentation
PT	16 s
APTT	47 s
Fibrinogen	1.5 g/l
TT	36 s
FDPs	1:1240
Sodium	134 mmol/l
Potassium	5.2 mmol/l
Urea	26 mmol/l
Creatinine	364 µmol/l
Urine microscopy	blood++, protein++

a) What is the likely diagnosis?

81

	Sat O_2(%)	Press (mmHg)
mRA		Mean 14
PA		27/12
PACW		Mean 24
Femoral artery	96	

This patient has a pansystolic murmur which developed 3 days after a myocardial infarction. There is a Swan–Ganz catheter in place. A femoral blood sample shows arterial saturation.

a) Can the patient lie flat?

b) What two diagnoses must be differentiated?

c) What simple measurement can be made without further cannulation to distinguish between these?

d) What effect will inspiration have on the murmur?

82 A 50 year old man was unable to work because of lethargy and depression. He was hypertensive and had mild angina. One year before he had been involved in a road traffic accident and sustained a head injury. He was pursuing an insurance claim and attributed his symptoms to anxiety. His medication was methyldopa 250 mg b.d., Moduretic two tablets daily and GTN p.r.n.

On examination he was pale, had thinning of his frontal hair and eyebrows and had lost most of his axillary and pubic hair. His neck, heart and lungs were normal. BP lying 120/70 mmHg, standing 105/60 mmHg. Neurological examination was normal apart from slow relaxation of his ankle jerks.

Investigations:

Hb	13 g/dl
WBC	$9 \times 10^9/l$
ESR	10 mm in the first hour
Sodium	126 mmol/l
Potassium	3.8 mmol/l
Urea	6 mmol/l
Albumin	40 g/l
Aspartate amino-transferase	30 iu/l
Alkaline phosphatase	100 iu/l
Bilirubin	5.5 μmol/l
Chest X-ray	normal
ECG	small voltage complexes
T4	50 nmol/l, TSH 1.0 mU/l
Anti microsomal antibodies	+1/1250

a) What is the diagnosis?

b) What investigations would you suggest?

c) What treatment and advice would you give him about his condition?

83 A 15 year old girl presents with a 2-month history of fatigue. She commenced her periods 18 months previously and these have recently become heavy. On three occasions in the past her mother has commented that she 'looks yellow'. Her father, who no longer lives at home, was diagnosed in his youth as having recurrent anaemia. She has no siblings and is on no medication. On examination she is pale and abdominal examination reveals 2 cm splenomegaly.

Investigations:

Hb	6.6 g/dl
WBC	$8.4 \times 10^9/l$
Platelets	$385 \times 10^9/l$
Reticulocytosis	10%
Direct Coomb's test	negative
Sodium	141 mmol/l
Potassium	4.9 mmol/l
Urea	4.3 mmol/l
Bilirubin	38 μmol/l
Aspartate transaminase	69 iu/l
Alkaline phosphatase	119 iu/l
Haptoglobins	not detected
Urinary haemosiderin	absent

a) What is the likely diagnosis and how would you investigate further?

84 A 38 year old woman presents with a 2-day history of a painful swollen right leg. Eight years previously she had had a similar episode which spontaneously resolved. Three weeks previously she had had an upper respiratory tract infection for which she was prescribed amoxycillin by her family doctor. Over the previous 3 years she had noticed the occasional passing of dark urine, particularly first thing in the morning. This, coupled with a complaint of intermittent colicky abdominal pain, led her family doctor to perform an IVU and abdominal ultrasound 1 year ago, both of which were normal. Her father died at the age of 50 from a cerebrovascular accident and there is a strong family history of hypertension. She smokes 20 cigarettes a day, drinks no alcohol and is on no regular medication.

On examination she is pyrexial 38.2°C, normotensive and has a tense, erythematous, painful, swollen left calf.

Investigations:

Hb	8.9 g/dl
WBC	2.3 × 10⁹/l (40% neutrophils)
Platelets	43 × 10⁹/l
Sodium	143 mmol/l
Potassium	3.6 mmol/l
Urea	4.3 mmol/l
Bilirubin	12 µmol/l
Aspartate amino-transferase	32 iu/l
Alkaline phosphatase	124 iu/l
PT	12 s
APTT	37 s
Fibrinogen	2.6 g/l
Thrombin time	15 s

a) What is the likely diagnosis?

b) How would you confirm your diagnosis?

85 A 28 year old man with a 6-year history of Crohn's disease has a 6-month history of frequent offensive loose stools and weight loss of 9 kg. General examination is unremarkable and sigmoidoscopy shows normal mucosa to the rectosigmoid junction, with views partially obscured by loose faeces and mucus.

Investigations:

Sodium	136 mmol/l
Potassium	4.2 mmol/l
Urea	4.4 mmol/l
Creatinine	110 μmol/l
Calcium	2.18 mmol/l
Albumin	34 g/l
Hb	13.2 g/dl
MCV	106 fl
PTT	22 s
3 day faecal fat	22 mmol/24 hours
Vit B_{12}	64 ng/l

Schilling test:
24 hr urine radioactivity minus IF: low
24 hr urine radioactivity plus IF: low
24 hr urine vol 1220 mls
24 hr urine creatinine 7.8 g/l

$^{14}CO_2$ breath test ^{14}C in breath – high
 ^{14}C in faeces – low

What is the likely explanation for the results of the Schilling test?

86A A 36 year old Indian man has the following blood count on a routine check-up:

Hb	12.8 g/dl
MCV	64 fl
MCH	24 pg
MCHC	26 g/dl
WBC	5.6 × 10^9/l
Platelets	237 × 10^9/l
Hb electrophoresis	A A2 F

a) What is the cause of the haematological abnormalities?
b) What action would you take?

86B The following results are obtained in a 32 year old woman with galactorrhoea:

Sodium	136 mmol/l
Potassium	5.5 mmol/l
Bicarbonate	18 mmol/l
Calcium (corrected)	2.04 mmol/l
Hb	8.6 g/dl
MCV	92 fl
MCH	32 pg
T4	48 nmol/l
TSH	2.4 mU/l

a) What is this woman's primary condition?

87 A 64 year old Somali woman has a 6-month history of 2-stone weight loss and episodic severe colicky abdominal pain, not associated with meals, posture or bowel habit. The following investigations are performed:

Sodium	125 mmol/l
Potassium	6.4 mmol/l
Urea	14 mmol/l
Calcium	2.76 mmol/l
Glucose	3.3 mmol/l
T4	34 nmol/l
TSH	24 mU/l
Thyroid microsomal antibodies	not detected

a) What is the diagnosis?

b) What treatment is indicated for the endocrine abnormalities?

88 This is the report of an exercise tolerance test. Standard
Bruce protocol was used. The test was terminated at
5 minutes 22 seconds with chest pain.

a) What is the most likely pathology underlying this change?

b) The patient's resting blood pressure on no treatment is
110/70. What other condition must be considered?

c) What 2 important investigations should be considered?

Pre-exercise ECG   0.75 cm = 1 mV

Post-exercise ECG   0.75 cm = 1 mV

89A A 36 year old man presents with a sudden history of lower abdominal pain and weakness of the right leg. Eight years previously he had had an aortic valve replacement. Since then he has been maintained on warfarin and propranolol until 2 weeks prior to presentation when the propranolol had been changed to a different antiarrhythmic agent. On examination he is in pain. In the cardiovascular system he has an ejection systolic murmur maximal at the left sternal edge.
Neurologically he has a flaccid right leg with loss of sensation to pin-prick and light touch over the lateral aspect of the right thigh. The right patellar reflex is absent.

Investigations:

Hb	9.6 g/dl
WBC	7.4 × 10^9/l
Platelets	374 × 10^9/l
Sodium	145 mmol/l
Potassium	4 mmol/l
Urea	4.7 mmol/l
Bilirubin	23 µmol/l
Aspartate amino-transferase	25 iu/l
Alkaline phosphatase	123 iu/l
PT	93 s
APTT	48 s
Fibrinogen	3.1 g/l

a) What is the likely diagnosis and how would you treat this man?

89B A 43 year old woman presents with a history of increasing tiredness. Seven years previously she was successfully treated with combined chemotherapy and radiotherapy for stage IV Hodgkin's disease.

Investigations:

Hb	10.2 g/dl
WBC	3.4 × 10^9/l neutrophils 34%, Pelger cells and occasional blasts
Platelets	49 × 10^9/l
MCV	108 fl

a) What is the likely cause of her anaemia?

Question 90

90 This is the ECG of a 14 year old boy who has recurrent dizzy
spells.
a) What is the diagnosis?
b) What two arrhythmias may underlie the dizzy spells? What
is the danger of the less common of the two?
c) Give 3 other causes of a positive R-wave in lead V1.

Limb leads (see overleaf for Chest leads).

V_1 V_4

V_2 V_5

V_3 V_6

Chest leads

91A A 75 year old man presents with tiredness. On examination he is pale, has widespread lymphadenopathy and a 6 cm spleen.

Investigations:

Hb	7.6 g/dl
WBC	28 × 10⁹/l – 92% lymphocytes
Platelet	52 × 10⁹/l
Blood film	polychromasia and spherocytes
Reticulocytes	8%
Serum haptoglobins	undetected

a) What is the likely diagnosis?

b) How would you confirm your diagnosis?

91B Investigations from a 5 year old child:

PT	14 s
APPT	80 s
TT	12 s
Fibrinogen	3.5 g
Bleeding time	7 minutes

a) What is the likely diagnosis?

b) What are the likely complications?

92 A 59 year old woman presents to outpatients with increasing tiredness and thirst. She has frequent epigastric pain and has woken on 3 occasions in the night with such pain in the last week.

Investigations:

Hb	11.3 g/dl
WBC	$6.4 \times 10^9/l$
Platelets	$264 \times 10^9/l$
ESR	9 mm in the first hour
Sodium	136 mmol/l
Potassium	4.3 mmol/l
Urea	11.5 mmol/l
Creatinine	140 μmol/l
Calcium	3.25 mmol/l
Phosphate	0.72 mmol/l
Chloride	117 mmol/l
Bicarbonate	12 mmol/l
Alkaline phosphatase	170 iu/l
Albumin	40 g/l

a) What is the likely diagnosis? What is the significance of the epigastric pain?

b) How do these patients usually present?

c) How would you confirm your diagnosis?

d) Give a differential diagnosis.

93 A 40 year old woman presents with a 3-month history of polyarthralgia and progressive difficulty climbing stairs.

Investigations:

Hb	13 g/dl
WBC	$5 \times 10^9/l$
Platelets	$250 \times 10^9/l$
ESR	36 mm in the first hour
Urea	5 mmol/l
Creatinine	130 mmol/l
Albumin	40 g/l
Aspartate amino-transferase	65 iu/l
Bilirubin	14 µmol/l
Alkaline phosphatase	120 iu/l
IgG	28 g/l
T4	80 nmol/l
Closed muscle biopsy	Normal

EMG Spontaneous fibrillation, high-frequency repetitive discharges and polyphasic short small motor-unit potentials

a) What is the most likely diagnosis?

94 a) Why was this glucose tolerance test performed on this 60 year old man?

b) What conclusions may be drawn from it?

Time	Blood glucose	Growth hormone
min	mmol/l	ng/l
0	8	12
30	13	13
60	16	11
90	12	12
120	10	12.5

Growth hormone normal basal value <5 iu/l

95A A 62 year old man has been treated with twice weekly haemodialysis for chronic renal failure secondary to reflux nephropathy. A subtotal parathyroidectomy had successfully been performed 3 years earlier.

He complains of aching lower back pain and his wife reminds him that he has become increasingly forgetful of late. Medication includes iron and folic acid supplements, aluminium hydroxide and nifedipine.

Investigations:

Sodium	140 mmol/l
Potassium	4.5 mmol/l
Urea	24 mmol/l
Creatinine	560 μmol/l
Calcium	2.4 mmol/l
Phosphate	1.4 mmol/l
Alkaline phosphatase	120 iu/l
PTH	undetectable
Radiological survey	mild demineralisation only

a) What is the likely diagnosis?
b) What treatment would you recommend?

95B A 10 year old boy is admitted for investigation. His mother has noted that he has become progressively clumsy. On examination he is alert and orientated. Abnormal findings were a right-sided intention tremor and right-sided nystagmus.

Investigations:

Hb	16 g/dl
WBC	6 × 10⁹/l
Platelets	225 × 10⁹/l
PCV	55%
Urea and electrolytes	normal

a) The history and signs point to a diagnosis in which part of the brain?
b) Give one unifying diagnosis.

96 A 75 year old man is found lying on the floor of his house. On admission he is hypothermic, bradycardic, and peripherally shut down. Electrocardiogram shows sinus bradycardia with ST elevation in leads II, III and AVF. Emergency electrolytes show:

Sodium   135 mmol/l
Potassium   5.0 mmol/l
Bicarbonate 12 mmol/l
Chloride   100 mmol/l
Urea   7.5 mmol/l

a) Comment on the biochemistry and how you would confirm your diagnosis.

97 This is the M-mode echocardiogram of a 40 year old woman.
a) What disease causes this valve lesion?
b) What is structure A?
c) Describe 2 abnormalities of structure B.
d) What physical sign would coincide with line C?

98 A 60 year old man was admitted with a 4-day history of fever, myalgias and headache. Two days before admission the patient had developed abdominal pain and had 3 loose stools. The GP was called by his wife when he became disorientated and confused. He had had no serious illnesses in the past and took no regular medication. He was a non-smoker and drank approximately one pint of beer a day.

Examination: Temperature 40°C; pulse 100 regular, BP 120/70 mmHg, respiration rate 24/min. The patient was clinically disorientated but specific examination of the nervous system was normal apart from mild neck stiffness. There was no anaemia, cyanosis, rash, lymphadenopathy or jaundice. Crackles were heard at his right base and in the left mid-zone. Examination of the heart was normal. There was diffuse abdominal tenderness and his liver edge could be felt two finger-breadths below the costal margin in the mid-clavicular line.

Investigations:

Hb	13.5 g/dl
WBC	15 × 10⁹/l – neutrophils 95%, lymphocytes 4 %
Platelets	300 × 10⁹/l
ESR	110 mm in the first hour
Sodium	127 mmol/l
Potassium	3.8 mmol/l
Urea	10.0 mmol/l
Creatinine	110 μmol/l
Albumin	38 g/l
Calcium	1.9 mmol/l
Phosphate	0.8 mmol/l
Bilirubin	14 μmol/l
Aspartate transaminase	80 iu/l
Alkaline phosphatase	200 iu/l
Glucose	5.0 mmol/l
pH	7.4
pO₂	9.0 kPa
pCO₂	4.0 kPa
Chest X-ray	increased shadowing in the right base and a small pleural effusion
CSF	Glucose 4.0 mmol/l, protein 0.8 g/l, <3 WBC/mm³ No bacteria seen

Routine cultures of blood, urine and CSF, and throat washings and stool were negative. The patient was started on intravenous amoxycillin but continued to deteriorate.

a) What is the most likely diagnosis?

b) How would you confirm your diagnosis?

c) How would you treat this patient?

99 A 60 year old woman presented with abdominal pain. She had been unwell for 2–3 weeks and felt 'weak'. For 3 weeks she had had intermittent sharp pains in her left upper quadrant and more recently a dull ache in her left iliac fossa. A week before admission she developed night sweats. There had been several episodes when she had become dizzy and confused and on one occasion she had lost vision in her left eye. She had a number of vague rheumatic symptoms but no early morning stiffness, headaches or jaw claudication. In the past she had had a hysterectomy and a cholecystectomy. She took no regular medication. There was no family history of significant disease.

Temperature 39°C, pulse 120, BP 140/60 mmHg, respiratory rate 40/min. She had no rash, lymphadenopathy or clubbing. Two small conjunctival haemorrhages were visible. Examination of her respiratory system was unremarkable. Her heart sounds were normal; a soft pansystolic murmur could be heard only at the apex. There was a tender pulsatile mass in the left iliac fossa and the spleen was palpable and tender. Neurological examination was normal. The peripheral pulses were present and equal. There were no bruits.

Investigations:

Hb	11 g/dl
WBC	8.0 × 10⁹/l
Platelets	300 × 10⁹/l
ESR	50 mm in the first hour
Sodium	140 mmol/l
Potassium	4.0 mmol/l
Urea	9 mmol/l
Creatinine	90 μmol/l
Albumin	30 g/l
Bilirubin	8.0 μmol/l
Aspartate amino-transferase	40 iu/l
Alkaline phosphatase	140 iu/l
Calcium	2.0 mmol/l
Chest X-ray and abdominal X-rays	normal
ECG	sinus tachycardia
Urinalysis	protein +; blood + no casts seen

An ultrasound of the abdomen showed a large spleen with wedge-shaped areas of increased density.

a) What is the most likely diagnosis?
b) Suggest three investigations.

100 An anxious 20 year old woman presented with mild shortness
of breath on exertion, which had come on gradually over
several months. The symptoms were intermittent but seemed to
be worse in the evening. Her husband complained that during
the episodes she appeared depressed and her speech was
slurred. She had been treated for depression in the past and
recently had been started on lorazepam by her GP for anxiety.

On examination in outpatients she looked very well. There
was no anaemia, cyanosis, clubbing, jaundice or oedema.
Examination of her respiratory and cardiovascular system was
normal. Abdominal examination was normal. The cranial nerves,
muscle tone, power, coordination and tendon reflexes were
normal. Sensation was intact.

Investigations:

FBC	normal
ESR	20 mm in the first hour
Electrolytes and liver function tests	normal
Chest X-ray	normal
Lung function tests	normal

a) What is the most likely diagnosis?

b) What tests would you perform?

101 Part 1 This is the M-mode echocardiograph at the level of mid left ventricle. Centimetre marks are shown.

Part 2 This is the apical doppler signal across the aortic valve.

ECG

Phonograph

A

Doppler signal

a) What abnormality is demonstrated in the left ventricle?
b) What is A on the phonocardiogram?
c) During which phase of the cardiac cycle is the dominant doppler signal shown and is it towards or away from the apex?
d) What is the cause of the left ventricular abnormality?

102 A 63 year old man who lived alone was referred with a short history of confusion and urinary incontinence. He had mild maturity-onset diabetes controlled by diet alone and was hypertensive. Regular treatment included bendrofluazide and propranolol 40 mg b.d. Eighteen months ago he had had meningococcal meningitis which had responded well to penicillin. He had no history of head injury and no history of epilepsy. He was a lifelong non-smoker and did not drink alcohol. Although he lived alone he had good support from his daughter who lived in the same street and provided his meals.

Temperature was 37°C, pulse 70 regular, BP 140/70 mmHg. On examination he was alert and orientated in person but not in time or location. He was unable to remember simple sentences and confabulated. His memory of recent events was poor. He was unable to perform simple arithmetic. There was no evidence of dysphasia, apraxia, or agnosia. There was no neck stiffness and no papilloedema. The cranial nerves were normal; examination of limbs revealed no motor or sensory signs. Coordination in his lower limbs was poor; he had a wide-based, fixed-footed gait and tended to fall unless he had assistance.

Examination of his chest and abdomen was unremarkable.

Investigations:

Urinalysis	normal
Sodium	137 mmol/l
Potassium	3.7 mmol/l
Urea	7 mmol/l
Calcium	2.3 mmol/l
Albumin	38 g/l
Total protein	75 g/l
Urate	6.0 mmol/l
WBC	7×10^9/l
Platelets	400×10^9/l
ESR	30 mm in the first hour
B_{12} and folate	normal
CRP	8 mg/l
VDRL	neg
T4	90 nmol/l
TSH	2.0 mU/l
CXR and skull X-ray	normal

a) What is the most likely diagnosis?

b) What is the treatment and what complications may follow?

103 A young man is admitted because he is breathless.

PEFR 200 l/min
Blood gases air
pH 7.5 ↑
pO₂ 9 kPa
pCO₂ 3.5 kPa
Bicarbonate 12 mmol/l

a) What are the abnormalities and how would you correct them?

Later his blood gases on 40% oxygen are:

pH 7.28
pO₂ 8 kPa
pCO₂ 6.5 ↑
Bicarbonate 17 mmol/l

b) What has happened? Give a differential diagnosis. What treatment would you consider?

104 This is an M-mode echocardiogram through the aortic root (space A).

a) What is B?

b) What is causing B?

c) What is C and is it normal?

d) The underlying disease is rheumatic heart disease – what can be deduced about the mitral valve?

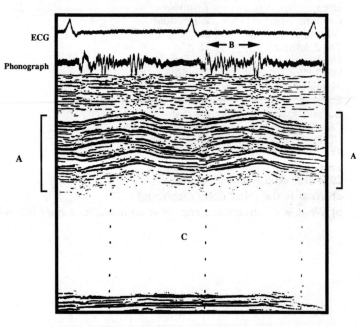

105 A 12 year old boy developed recurrent upper abdominal pain and intermittent diarrhoea after returning from a short holiday with his school to Leningrad. The stools were bulky, pale and offensive. He had no fever and had an excellent appetite. In the past he had had whooping cough and since then had regular attacks of bronchitis during the winter, but was able to play games and had little time off school.
On examination he had no rash, anaemia, clubbing, lymphadenopathy or jaundice. His height was on the 50th centile and weight 60% of that predicted for an average boy of his age. His two other siblings were both within the normal range. Examination of the cardiovascular system was normal. Examination of the chest revealed crackles at his left base and right mid-zone. On palpation his abdomen was soft and there was no organomegaly. His right colon was easily palpable and loaded with faeces. Examination of the CNS was normal.

Investigations:

Hb	13 g/dl
WBC	9×10^9/l
Platelets	400×10^9/l
ESR	50 mm in the first hour
Sodium	137 mmol/l
Potassium	4.1 mmol/l
Urea	6 mmol/l
Albumin	25 g/l
Total protein	70 g/l
B$_{12}$	300 ng/l
Folate	2 µg/l
Iron	17 µmol/l
TIBC	50 µmol/l
Faecal fat excretion	28 mmol/l

CXR small patches of atelectasis in the left base. AXR a dilated colon loaded with faeces.

a) What is the most likely diagnosis?

b) What investigations would you request?

106 A 65 year old man was reviewed in clinic. He complained of increased shortness of breath on exertion and was breathless walking up two flights of stairs. Recently he had felt increasingly tired, with myalgia and pain in a number of his joints but no swelling or stiffness. His GP had increased his dose of frusemide without apparent benefit. Seven years previously he had had aortic valve replacement for aortic regurgitation. A second Starr–Edwards prosthesis was inserted 3 years after an episode of infective endocarditis. Two years later he had developed atrial fibrillation which was controlled by digoxin and verapamil; on examination, crepitations were heard in his lung bases and 40 mg of frusemide was started. A right heart catheter was passed and a normal wedge pressure recorded. An echocardiogram indicated that the aortic prosthesis was functioning well and the other heart valves were normal. The atrial fibrillation had become difficult to control with digoxin and verapamil 6 months ago and they had been replaced with amiodarone, with marked symptomatic improvement. He was a lifelong non-smoker and had no exposure to occupational dusts or fumes.

Now on examination he was warm but peripherally cyanosed. Pulse 80 irregularly irregular, blood pressure 110/70, JVP visible. The cardiac apex beat was not palpable and there were no abnormal heaves or thrills. Auscultation revealed prosthetic heart sounds only. There were fine inspiratory crackles audible in the lower zones of both lungs.

A chest X-ray showed diffuse linear shadowing in both lower zones. The ECG had not changed from previous visits and showed atrial fibrillation with left bundle branch block.

Investigations:

Hb	15 g/l
WBC	8×10^9/l
Platelets	300×10^9/l
ESR	80 mm in the first hour
Sodium	135 mmol/l
Potassium	3.5 mmol/l
Urea	12 mmol/l
Creatinine	90 μmol/l
Albumin	45 g/l
Total protein	90 g/l
Aspartate transaminase	40 iu/l
Alkaline phosphatase	120 iu/l
Bilirubin	10 μmol/l
Rheumatoid factor	1/80
ANA positive	1/40
PEFR	450
FEV1	90%
FVC	70%

a) What is the most likely cause of the breathlessness?
b) What 3 investigations would you arrange?

107 This patient has recurrent syncope.
- **a)** Identify three abnormalities.
- **b)** How is the ventricular mass depolarised?
- **c)** What underlies the syncope and what treatment is indicated?

Limb leads (see overleaf for Chest leads.)

Chest leads

20 mm/sec; 0.8 cm/mV

108 A woman aged 27 years in the 30th week of her first pregnancy, complained of tiredness and breathlessness on exertion. She had had no chest pain, cough or haemoptysis but had had mild facial flushing. She had no history of foreign travel and was not exposed to hazardous fumes in the factory where she worked. There was no family history of illness. She had not had any serious illnesses in the past. She was a non-smoker who drank little alcohol and had never abused drugs. She had taken the oral contraceptive pill for 8 years before deciding to become pregnant.

On examination, she looked pale; her hands and feet were cold and cyanosed. She was not anaemic or clubbed. Pulse of 90, blood pressure 90/65 mmHg with no elevation of the jugular venous pressure. She had a palpable right ventricular heave. On auscultation a loud pulmonary second sound and a soft fourth heart sound could be heard. Her lung fields were clear. There was mild pitting oedema in both ankles.

Investigations:

Hb	14 g/dl
WBC	5.6 × 10⁹/l
Platelets	400 × 10⁹/l
Sodium	139 mmol/l
Potassium	3.9 mmol/l
Urea	5.9 mmol/l
Albumin	45 g/l
Total protein	75 g/l
Aspartate transaminase	36 iu/l
Alkaline phosphatase	120 iu/l
Bilirubin	4.5 μmol/l
ESR	30 mm in the first hour
CRP	10 mg/l
T4	80 nmol/l
TSH	2.0 mU/l

FEV_1 90%, FVC 100%, TLCO 95%, VA 90%, KCO 95%
CXR prominent pulmonary arteries, lung fields clear.

a) Give the two differential diagnoses.

b) What 4 investigations would you request?

109A A 48 year old woman was referred to casualty with headaches and somnolence. The headaches were diffuse and were worse on waking. The symptoms had begun 5 days earlier following an influenza-like illness. She had had mild breathlessness on exertion for several years which she attributed to her increasing weight and smoking 20 cigarettes per day. She had no serious medical problems in the past and took no regular medication.

On examination she was alert, had no anaemia or cyanosis. Her weight was 125 kg. Examination of her cardiorespiratory system was normal. Examination of her central nervous system was normal. There was no neck stiffness and her fundi were clear.

Investigations:

CXR	normal
Blood gases	air
pH	7.4
pO_2	10.5 kPa
pCO_2	6.5 kPa
Bicarbonate	32 mmol/l

a) What is the diagnosis?

b) What treatment would you suggest?

109B A 26 year old woman attends her GP with cystitis, for which he prescribes an empirical course of trimethoprim. Five days later her symptoms persist and she complains of nausea and occasional vomiting. In addition to sending an MSU for culture, the GP checks her serum biochemistry, the results of which are:

Sodium	138 mmol/l
Potassium	4.4 mmol/l
Bicarbonate	21 mmol/l
Urea	5.6 mmol/l
Creatinine	183 µmol/l

a) What is the likely explanation for the patient's biochemical abnormality?

110 A 40 year old man was sent to the casualty department from a local hostel for the homeless after being found lying on the floor, confused and smelling strongly of alcohol. Only a limited history was available from the patient; the warden, who knew him well, thought he had been feeling unwell for several weeks and had had a recent course of antibiotics prescribed by the GP.

Examination in casualty showed a left-sided scalp laceration with extensive bruising. Neurological examination was normal. Apart from a temperature of 38°C, overnight observations were satisfactory. He awoke the next day feeling listless and complaining of a dull headache and nausea. Later he began vomiting and then collapsed and was incontinent. Further neurological examination revealed weakness down the right side, reduced tone and a right extensor plantar response.

Investigations:

Hb	12.9 g/l
WBC	10 × 10⁹/l – mild neutrophilia
Platelets	300 × 10⁹/l
Sodium	130 mmol/l
Potassium	3.8 mmol/l
Urea	8 mmol/l
Glucose	8 mmol/l
ESR	55 mm in the first hour
CRP	35 mg/l
Protein electrophoresis	increased gamma globulins
Urinalysis	normal
CXR	old apical calcification
Skull X-rays	normal
CT head scan	small left parietal infarct

Lumbar puncture – difficult

Lymphocytes	300/mm³
Neutrophils	20/mm³
RBC	70 mm³
Protein	3 g/l
Glucose	2.5 mmol/l
Gram stain and ZN stain	no organisms

a) What is the most likely diagnosis?
b) What is the likely cause of his deterioration?

111A A 55 year old woman was found during the course of a routine medical examination to have a monoclonal band on protein electrophoresis.

Investigations:

IgG	20 g/l
IgM	0.8 g/l
IgA	2.5 g/l
Albumin	38 g/l
Calcium	2.4 mmol/l
Akaline phosphatase	125 iu/l
Hb	12.9 g/dl
WBC	$5.7 \times 10^9/l$
Platelets	$267 \times 10^9/l$
ESR	45 mm in the first hour
Bence-Jones protein	negative
Bone marrow	3% plasma cells
Radiographic survey	normal

a) What diagnosis would you attach to her?

b) How would you manage her?

111B A 45 year old smoker complains of tiredness and weakness.

Investigations:

Blood pressure	180/110 mmHg
Sodium	140 mmol/l
Potassium	2.8 mmol/l
Bicarbonate	32 mmol/l
Urea	5 mmol/l
Glucose	12 mmol/l

a) What is the probable diagnosis?

b) What 2 investigations would you perform to confirm your diagnosis?

112 A 70 year old man is admitted with exertional dyspnoea and bilateral leg oedema. He gives a 3-month history of bilateral numbness and tingling of the fingers.

Investigations:

Hb	11.8 g/dl
WBC	5 × 10⁹/l
Platelets	350 × 10⁹/l
ESR	98 mm in the first hour
Urea	8 mmol/l
Creatinine	130 mmol/l
Uric acid	0.5 mmol/l
Albumin	20 g/l
Alkaline phosphatase	100 iu/l
Aspartate aminotransferase	25 iu/l
Plasma electrophoresis	IgG monoclonal protein with immune paresis
24 hour protein excretion	8 g
ECG	low voltage complexes with 2:1 heart block

a) What is the likely underlying diagnosis?

b) Why is the patient short of breath and oedematous?

113 A 66 year old man has attended his GP with a 3-year history of late-onset asthma and more recent exertional angina and intermittent claudication. He attends the surgery with a 3-week history of mild dyspnoea on exertion. Examination confirms a moderate expiratory wheeze and a peak flow reading of 230 l/min is obtained. The GP prescribes a 1-week course of ampicillin in addition to his usual Ventolin inhaler. One week later the patient returns with no improvement. On examination, his temperature is 37.4°C. He has widespread expiratory wheezes. His blood pressure is 155/102. He has a number of purpuric lesions on his feet. The following investigations are performed:

Hb	12 g/dl
WBC	11.8×10^9/l
Neutrophils	7.2×10^9/l
Lymphocytes	1.4×10^9/l
Eosinophils	3×10^9/l
Urea	13.6 mmol/l
Creatinine	210 μmol/l
FEV 1	2.8 l
FVC	4.9 l
Urinalysis	Protein ++
	blood – non-haemolysed trace
Urine microscopy	20 white cells/hpf
	scanty granular casts.

a) What is the probable diagnosis?

b) What clinical features are suggestive of this diagnosis?

c) Give two other causes of renal impairment associated with eosinophilia.

114A The following results are obtained in a 72 year old smoker:

Sodium	119 mmol/l
Potassium	3.6 mmol/l
Blood uric acid	0.08 mmol/l
Urea	4.5 mmol/l
Glucose	5.2 mmol/l
Urinary sodium	54 mmol/l
Urinary osmolality	456 mmol/kg

a) What pathology is suggested by these results?

b) What are the three principles of treatment?

114B What investigation is indicated to explain this patient's
hyponatraemia?

Sodium	118 mmol/l
Potassium	4.3 mmol/l
Urea	4.8 mmol/l
Glucose	4.6 mmol/l
Plasma osmolality	284 mmol/kg
Albumin	24 g/l
24 hour urinary protein	7.8 g

115 **a)** This patient has had a pacemaker inserted for two separate
rhythm disturbances. What are they?

Limb leads

Chest leads   17.5 min/sec; 0.75 cm/mV

116 A 36 year old woman, weighing 60 kg, is admitted following a suspected overdose. No tablets are found at gastric lavage and salicylate and paracetamol are not detected in the plasma. She is admitted for observation. Eleven hours after admission the patient's condition deteriorates and she rapidly becomes unconscious, with a respiratory rate of 36/minute. The following results are obtained:

Sodium	136 mmol/l
Potassium	5.7 mmol/l
Glucose	4.8 mmol/l
Bicarbonate (standardized)	8 mmol/l
Anion gap	36
Base excess	−20
Lactate	high
Urinalysis	crystalluria
PTT	15 s

a) What is the patient's calculated total bicarbonate (HCO_{3-}) deficit?

b) What is the diagnosis? What further complications may occur?

c) What are the 3 principles of management?

117 The following results are obtained in a 27 year old woman undergoing investigation for hypertension:

Sodium	136 mmol/l
Potassium	3.4 mmol/l
Urea	6.8 mmol/l
Creatinine	127 μmol/l
Right renal vein renin	× 1.5 inferior vena cava renin level
Left renal vein renin	× 2 inferior vena cava renin level

a) What is the probable diagnosis?

b) What is the explanation for the observed renin measurements?

c) What is the treatment of choice?

36 hours following treatment, the patient's BP is 110/70 lying and 90/40 standing.

d) How do you explain the postural hypotension observed 36 hours after therapy?

118 The following results are obtained during investigation of a 64 year old patient with back pain, anaemia and an acute phase response:

Hb	9 g/dl
MCV	84 fl
WBC	6.8×10^9/l
Platelets	276×10^9/l
ESR	100 mm in the first hour
Sodium	136 mmol/l
Potassium	3.3 mmol/l
Urea	9.9 mmol/l
Creatinine	183 µmol/l
Bicarbonate	15 mmol/l
Chloride	109 mmol/l
Alkaline phosphatase	174 iu/l
Calcium (corrected)	2.8 mmol/l
Glucose	4.3 mmol/l
Urinalysis (early morning)	pH 5.2
	protein +++
	glucose ++

a) What is the diagnosis?

b) Why is the urine well acidified?

c) What diagnostic procedures are indicated?

d) What urine constituent is the likely cause of proteinuria?

119 A 54 year old man with adult polycystic kidney disease (APCKD), and stable chronic renal failure, attends his GP with a recent history of polyuria and polydypsia, and left loin pain. He is on no medications. The following investigations are performed:

Hb	11.3 g/dl
WBC	$6 \times 10^9/l$
Platelets	$270 \times 10^9/l$
Sodium	147 mmol/l
Potassium	4.2 mmol/l
Bicarbonate	18 mmol/l
Urea	39 μmol/l
Creatinine	408 mmol/l
Calcium	3.1 mmol/l
Albumin	34 g/l
Alkaline phosphatase	188 iu
Plasma glucose	6.5 mmol/l
[PTH] (C-terminal assay)	slight increase
1.25 (OH)$_2$ D	normal
Urinalysis	blood ++++, protein +
Radiographic survey	normal

a) Give 2 appropriate diagnostic procedures.

b) Give two explanations for the patient's haemoglobin concentration.

c) What is the significance of the [PTH] result?

120 The following results were obtained in a patient with severe loin pain:

Sodium	138 mmol/l
Potassium	2.5 mmol/l
Urea	3.8 mmol/l
Chloride	114 mmol/l
Anion gap	12
Urinary pH	6.1

a) What is the bicarbonate concentration?

b) What is the diagnosis? What is the cause of the loin pain?

121 A 43 year old depressed woman is admitted with an overdose. There is a number of different empty bottles of tablets in her bedroom, and it is not clear what she has taken. Aspirin or paracetamol seem the most likely possibilities.

a) What clinical features would suggest aspirin overdose?

b) What type of initial biochemical disturbance would be expected? How might this change?

c) Explain the mechanisms which produce the metabolic disturbances in this condition.

d) How do salicylate levels correlate with toxicity?

e) What is the treatment?

122 A 61 year old female hospital domestic presented with an 8-week history of shivering attacks, increasing shortness of breath and leg oedema. Appetite was decreased and she had lost 3 kg in weight over this period. Past medical history included a perforated peptic ulcer 20 years previously non-insulin-dependent diabetes mellitus. On admission she was taking glibenclamide 10 mg o/d. She was a non-smoker and drank 10 glasses of rum per week. Five months ago she returned from a 4-week visit to her birthplace on the island of St. Lucia.

On examination she was pyrexial 37.8°C, clinically pale. Pulse 90 regular, B.P. 130/85 mmHg. Normal sclerae, no lymphadenopathy. Normal heart sounds with an apical systolic ejection murmur. Decreased movement on the right side of the chest with dull percussion note, diminished tactile vocal fremitus and absent breath sounds. The abdomen was soft with no organomegaly and the rest of the examination was normal.

Investigations:

Hb	9 g/dl
MCV	85 fl
Sickle cell	negative
WBC	8.9×10^9/l – 87% neutrophils
Platelets	450×10^9/l
ESR	66 mm in the first hour
Iron	6.0 μmol/l
Transferrin	1.5 g/l
Sodium	140 mmol/l
Potassium	4.5 mmol/l
Urea	5 mmol/l
Creatinine	130 mmol/l
Total protein	65 g/l
Albumin	19 g/l
Aspartate amino-transferase	45 iu/l
Bilirubin	15 μmol/l
Alkaline phosphatase	160 iu/L1
PT	19.3 s
PTTK	43 s
Autoantibody screen	weak positive ANA
Blood cultures	*Streptococcus milleri*
Urine	normal
Chest X-ray	right pleural effusion
Pleural fluid	protein 62 g/l

a) What is the likely diagnosis and how would you confirm your diagnosis?

b) How would you manage the patient?

123 A 53 year old hypertensive diabetic man presented to casualty feeling acutely dizzy and vomiting, with difficulty in speaking and a 'peculiar feeling' in his right arm and leg, and the left side of his face.

a) What is the probable diagnosis?

b) What physical signs would you expect to elicit?

c) i) Where is the lesion and ii) which vessel supplies this area?

d) How can the clinical findings be related directly to specific regions in the brain?

124 A 23 year old woman attends her GP for contraceptive advice. Her blood pressure is found to be 158/98 mmHg and she has Grade I hypertensive retinal changes. One week later she is seen in a medical outpatients clinic. She has no personal or family history of note, and in particular no history of cardiac or renal disease. On direct questioning she admits to a 'viral illness' some weeks previously. She is not taking any prescribed or proprietary medications. On examination the registrar describes her appearance as 'thin and drawn', though she denies any weight loss. Her BP is 170/104 in both arms and there is no radiofemoral delay. The retinal changes are confirmed. There is no abdominal bruit. A Grade I ejection systolic murmur is noted at the base of the heart. The rest of the examination is normal.

The following investigations are performed in outpatients:

Hb	11.5 g/dl
WBC	7.6 × 10^9/l
Platelets	376 × 10^9/l
Sodium	138 mmol/l
Potassium	4.4 mmol/l
Bicarbonate	22 mmol/l
Urea	11.5 mmol/l
Creatinine	156 µmol/l
Glucose	6.9 mmol/l
Urinalysis	blood ++, protein ++

MSU 10^3 organisms mixed growth
Urine microscopy – 30 red cells/hpf, scanty granular casts
Antinuclear factor – 1/80 homogeneous pattern
C3 17% NHP (N >60%)
C4 69% NHP (N >60%)
CH50 67% NHP (N >60%)
ECG and CXR are normal.

The patient is admitted for further investigation.

a) Suggest a likely diagnosis. What non-invasive investigation may support your clinical diagnosis?

b) Give a differential diagnosis.

125 Opposite is a series of excerpts from a 24 hour tape (lead V1, p. 101).

a) What is demonstrated?

19 mm/sec; 0.75 cm/mV

I

II

III

126 A 28 year old asthmatic man is admitted from outpatients with a 3-week history of progressive lower limb swelling. The rest of his history is unremarkable and his only medications are a Ventolin inhaler, and a proprietary analgesic for a sporting injury sustained 5 weeks previously.

Examination confirms pitting oedema to the thighs. Blood pressure is 130/78 with no postural hypotension.

The following investigations are performed:

Sodium	139 mmol/l
Potassium	4.8 mmol/l
Urea	8.7 mmol/l
Creatinine	112 µmol/l
Albumin	22 g/l
Urinalysis	protein ++++, blood negative
24 hr urine protein	5.7 g

Renal biopsy – normal appearances on light microscopy, podocyte effacement on electron microscopy

The patient's weight on admission is 83 kg. His fluid intake is restricted to 1 l per day, he is given a low-salt diet, and is prescribed a loop diuretic and high-dose steroids. Eight days later his weight is 71 kg and his serum urea and creatinine are 32 and 170 respectively. Urinalysis shows 4+'s proteinuria and 3+'s of blood. He informs the nursing staff of bilateral loin ache. That afternoon he experiences a sudden onset of shortness of breath, and arterial blood gas analysis shows a pO_2 of 6.7 kPa and a pCO_2 of 3.3 kPa.

a) What is the initial diagnosis? Give two potential causes of the initial renal lesion.

b) What complication has occurred?

127 This is a routine ECG.
   a) What is the predominant rhythm in the 12 lead recordings?
   b) In the rhythm strip, is atrial depolarization normal?

Limb lead (see overleaf for Chest lead).

V_1

V_4

V_2

V_5

V_3

V_6

Chest lead

20 mm/sec; 0.8 cm/mV

128 A 63 year old man comes into A & E with a 2-day history of severe leg pains, and increasing difficulty in walking. He was previously well, but both he and his wife had 'flu 10 days earlier. On examination, he was apyrexial, pulse 90 SR, BP 120/70 mmHg, chest clear, RR 22; no neck stiffness, but both his arms and legs were weak, and no tendon reflexes could be elicited.

a) What is the diagnosis?

b) What investigation is required? What would the findings be? Give a differential diagnosis of these findings.

c) What are the principles of management?

d) Name two related neurological conditions.

129 A 27 year old man is admitted to casualty very pale and unwell. He has a history of 2–3 weeks' haemoptysis and increasing malaise, and during the 24 hours prior to admission he has noticed a fall in urine output, and blood in his urine.

On examination: pulse 130 sinus rhythm; BP 145/95 mmHg; JVP + 9cm; RR 24/min; scattered crackles in both lung fields on auscultation.

Investigations:

Hb	8.3 g/dl mildly hypochromic
WBC	11.8 × 10⁹/l
Platelets	621 × 10⁹/l
Clotting	normal
Sodium	136 mmol/l
Potassium	7.6 mmol/l
Urea	32.1 mmol/l
Creatinine	769 μmol/l
ECG	peaked T-waves
CXR	patchy interstitial shadowing both lungs
Urine dipstick	protein +++, blood +++

a) What is the likely diagnosis? What other questions would you ask?

b) What other tests should be performed urgently?

c) What is the immediate priority in this patient's management?

130A A 45 year old man presented to the rheumatology clinic with painful knees. Past medical history included meningococcal meningitis at the age of 20 and gonorrhoea at the age of 24. He had otherwise enjoyed good health until 2 years ago when he became impotent and this had led to marital difficulties. He smoked 20 cigarettes a day and drank 4 pints of beer per night when on leave in the United Kingdom.

On examination he looked well with a marked suntan, having recently returned from Saudi Arabia where he worked as an engineer. Marked crepitus was present in both knees. Testes were small and pubic hair sparse.

Investigations:

Hb	14 g/dl
WBC	5 × 10⁹/l
ESR	15 mm in the first hour
Urea and electrolytes	normal
Urine dipstick	glucose ++

a) What is the cause of the arthritis? What is the likely diagnosis?

b) How would you confirm your diagnosis?

130B A 57 year old woman is admitted following a collapse. She complains of recent difficulty in rising from her armchair. Her blood pressure is 168/108 with 8 mmHg systolic postural drop. She has recently been taking a proprietary analgesic for osteoarthritis. The following results are obtained:

Sodium	136 mmol/l
Potassium	6.8 mmol/l
Bicarbonate	16 mmol/l
Urea	17 mmol/l
Creatinine	270 µmol/l
Chloride	110 mmol/l
HbA1c	9%
Aldosterone	low
Urinalysis	protein +++

a) What is the underlying diagnosis?
b) What is the serum renin concentration likely to be?
c) What is the likely explanation for the collapse?
d) Give 2 possible causes of the lower limb weakness.

Answers

1 a) Fasting hypoglycaemia due to excess insulin secretion. With a blood glucose of 2.9 mmol/l, plasma insulin level should be <3 mU/l.

b) An insulinoma is the commonest cause of excess insulin secretion. The important differential diagnosis in this case is self-administration of insulin. The latter can be excluded by measurement of plasma-immunoreactive C-peptide which will be low in cases of exogenous insulin administration and high with an endogenous insulin source. Retroperitoneal fibrosarcoma and mesothelioma can also induce hypoglycaemia by secretion of insulin-like growth factors.

Spontaneous hypoglycaemia can be divided into 2 groups:
1) Fasting hypoglycaemia-symptoms occur at night, in the early morning or after a fast. This group can be subdivided into
i) Excess insulin production or self administration (no ketosis) e.g.
   Insulinoma
   Retroperitoneal fibrosarcoma
   Mesothelioma
ii) Non-insulin induced causes (ketonaemia is a feature) e.g.
   Liver failure
   Addison's disease, hypopituitarism
   Ethanol, sulphonylureas, aspirin, propranolol
   Septicaemia, malaria
   Autoimmune hypoglycaemia–insulin receptor autoantibodies
   End-stage renal disease
2) Post-prandial or reactive hypoglycaemia symptoms occur 2–4 hours after eating.

Insulinoma
One of the commonest causes of non-diabetic fasting-induced hypoglycaemia. These are tumours of the B cells and can occur in any part of the pancreas. The majority are benign and slow growing, but 10% are malignant.

Median age of presentation is the 5th decade. Patients typically present with drowsiness on waking which is relieved by eating. Other modes of presentation include fits, dizziness, diplopia and paraesthesiae. Patients may become obese as their calorie consumption increases in an attempt to avoid symptoms.

2 A
a) Blood drawn upstream from an intravenous dextrose infusion.

B
a) Failure to separate red blood cells from plasma. Glucose is utilized by the red cells, therefore is low. Potassium and phosphate are falsely high due to leakage from the red cells. The blood had been drawn on the previous evening.

C
a) The first sample was taken supine and the second after 20 minutes ambulation. A degree of haemoconcentration accompanies the erect posture as small water molecules enter the extravascular space. Haemoconcentration also accompanies prolonged stasis. Stasis however results in local hypoxia and acidosis which elevates the serum potassium concentration.

3 a) Ischaemic heart disease is the commonest cause of atrial arrhythmias.
b) Insertion of a pacemaker. Whatever the atrial rhythm there is atrioventricular (AV) nodal dysfunction with AV conduction disturbance.
c) Quinidine speeds the conduction through the AV node and can cause 1:1 conduction of atrial flutter with a ventricular rate of 300.

4 a) i) Reversible obstructive airways disease – presumably an infective exacerbation of asthma in this case. ii) (Variable) extrathoracic tracheal obstruction.

Note: C is a normal flow–volume loop.

The first flow–volume loop in the question is typical of severe obstructive airways disease. The normal expiratory limb in the second loop confirms that this must be reversible airways obstruction, i.e. asthma. The inspiratory limb of the second flow loop is abnormal. The MIF_{50} is the inspiratory flow rate at 50% of the vital capacity and in this instance is approximately half that expected. This confirms an extrathoracic tracheal obstruction which must be variable as the expiratory limb is unaffected. In the clinical context, this is likely to be a consequence of long-term intubation, with development of a tracheal stricture – this patient should have been managed with a tracheostomy. Other causes of extrathoracic tracheal obstruction include vocal cord palsies, malignancy and infective and inflammatory conditions, including Wegener's granulomatosis and syphilis. The other important pattern of flow–volume loop is that of a fixed intrathoracic tracheal obstruction, for example due to hilar malignancy, and in this instance both the inspiratory and expiratory limbs will be flattened.

C

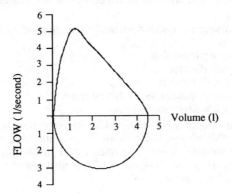

5 a) The most likely diagnosis is **acute rheumatic fever** and a **recent hepatitis A infection**.

b) Immediate management is bed rest, physiotherapy and acetyl/ salicylate as an anti-inflammatory agent (6-12 g/day) to achieve blood levels between 2.1 and 2.4 mmol/l. The dramatic response of the arthritis to salicylate therapy is characteristic. Oral penicillin 125–250 mg b.d. should be taken until the age of 20 years in all patients who have had carditis, to decrease the risk of a further attack of rheumatic fever. Daily oral penicillin or monthly intramuscular penicillin should be continued in adults who continue to be exposed to young children. There is no evidence that salicylates or steroids influence the prognosis.

She fulfils the **Duckett Jones criteria** for acute rheumatic fever, i.e. two major criteria or one major and two minor criteria plus evidence of a recent streptoccocal infection.

Major criteria of rheumatic fever include polyarthritis, carditis, erythema marginatum, subcutaneous nodules (Ashoff) and chorea.

Minor criteria include previous rheumatic fever, fever, arthralgia, raised ESR and prolonged P–R interval.

Evidence of recent group A streptococcal infection includes i) isolation of haemolytic streptococci from a throat swab, ii) rising antibody titre and iii) recent scarlet fever.

The differential diagnosis of rheumatic fever includes:

1) Rubella
2) Still's disease – childhood onset rheumatoid arthritis,
3) Hepatitis
4) Infective endocarditis
5) Sickle cell disease
6) Gonococcal arthritis
7) Malignancy–leukaemia or lymphoma
8) Familial Mediterranean Fever

The infectious hepatitis A acquired in Pakistan had settled before the onset of this illness (note there is no significant change in the hepatitis A antibody titres). The raised AST is caused by the rheumatic fever and the elevation of the enzyme is a measure of the severity of the attack.

6A a) The diagnosis is **pyschogenic polydipsia** (high 24 hour urine volumes). She is normovolaemic, as assessed by physical examination, and is hypotonic and hyponatraemic. This can only be caused by excess water in the extracellular space. The possibilities are ADH-dependent water retention, ADH-independent water retention (e.g. in chronic renal failure) or excess water intake. In the case of neurogenic diabetes insipidus the plasma osmolality and sodium are usually normal provided water is freely available.

b) In psychogenic polydipsia the ADH is appropriately low. If there is difficulty in distinguishing between neurogenic diabetes insipidus and psychogenic polydipsia, a water deprivation test should be performed with serial measurement of weight, plasma and urine osmolality and plasma ADH. The plasma osmolality should rise to above 290 mmol/l (to ensure an adequate stimulus for ADH secretion); in the case of true diabetes insipidus the urine osmolality will not increase appropriately. Desmopressin (an analogue of ADH) is then given; a rise in the osmolality of the urine will be seen with neurogenic diabetes insipidus but not with nephrogenic diabetes insipidus. In nephrogenic diabetes insipidus there is end-organ resistance to ADH (ADH levels typically normal). In some cases of psychogenic polydipsia the results of the water deprivation test may be difficult to interpret. This may be resolved by an infusion of hypertonic saline with serial measurements of plasma and urine osmolalities, along with plasma ADH levels and urine volumes.

6B a) Suprapubic bladder aspiration.
The urine sample contains numerous epithelial cells and a mixed-bacterial flora of oral commensals, strongly suggesting that the urine had been contaminated. On detailed examination of the mucosal cavity a laceration was seen on the inside of the cheek. The patient admitted that the injury was self-inflicted and that he had been spitting blood into his urine.

7A **a)** Hypocalcaemia leads to increased neuromuscular excitability, resulting in paraesthesiae of the extremities and circumoral areas, tetany, muscle cramps and fits.
Chvostek's test – tapping the facial nerve – may elicit a twitch. Trousseau's sign – inflation of a sphygmomanometer cuff for 3 minutes above the diastolic pressure – may elicit carpopedal spasm.

b) **Hypomagnesaemia** subsequent to *cis*-platinum therapy. Hypomagnesaemia occurs in approximately 50% of patients treated with *cis*-platinum as a result of renal magnesium loss. Hypomagnesaemia results in hypocalcaemia due to inhibition of parathyroid hormone release and impaired end-organ response to parathyroid hormone.
The patient should be given intravenous magnesium sulphate until magnesium levels normalize.

7B **a)** **Congestive cardiac failure**
b) The biochemical picture of low serum sodium, low potassium, high bicarbonate and elevated urea is explained by the secondary hypoaldosteronism that complicates severe congestive cardiac failure. Note that although serum sodium levels are low, total body serum sodium levels are high. The hypoalbuminaemia is explained by the protein-losing enteropathy which may complicate such a picture with a grossly oedematous intestinal mucosa. Oral drugs are often ineffective in such cases due to decreased absorption and drugs need to be given intravenously.

8 a) i) Recurrent lymphoma
  ii) Opportunistic infection – patient is immunosuppressed
      (particularly with *Pneumocystis carinii*)
  iii) Hepatic abscess
b) i) Bronchoscopy with washings and transbronchial biopsy
  ii) Ultrasound or CT scan of abdomen
  iii) Liver biopsy

Hodgkin's disease (Thomas Hodgkin 1832) is commoner overall in males, with two age peaks from 15–25 and 55–75 years of age. The disease is characterized by the presence of Reed–Sternberg cells. Four histological variants are described: i) lymphocyte predominant (10–15% – overall have the best prognosis); ii) mixed cellularity (20–40%); iii) lymphocyte depleted (5–15%), and iv) nodular sclerosing (20–50%). Clinically, patients present with enlarged lymph nodes (usually neck or axilla) or a mediastinal mass on chest X-ray. Twenty-five percent of patients have constitutional or B symptoms of pruritus, fever, alcohol-induced pain and >10% weight loss. Staging is according to the Ann Arbor classification – Stage I: A single lymph node or a single extralymphatic organ or site. Stage II: Two or more lymph node regions or an extranodal site and lymph nodes, on the same side of the diaphragm. Stage III: Nodes on both sides of the diaphragm, with or without splenic involvement. Stage IV: Diffuse involvement of one or more extralymphatic sites, with or without lymphadenopathy.

Treatment, broadly, is mantle or inverted Y radiotherapy for Stages I and II disease (unless bulky). Stage III and IV disease, along with bulky stage II disease are treated with combination chemotherapy using four drugs – the usual first choice being LOPP (chlorambucil, vincristine, procarbazine and prednisolone). Five-year survival without treatment is 10%, now it is 70–80% for all stages. Early stage, youth, the absence of B symptoms and good prognostic histology bode best.

The disease caused by *Pneumocystis carinii* is an extensive pneumonitis found almost exclusively in the immunosuppressed or immunodeficient host. Pathologically the disease is characterized by an extensive desquamative alveolitis. The organisms are clustered in the alveolar lumen. The 'foamy exudate' formerly described represents unstained clusters of cysts and alveolar cells with cytoplasmic vacuoles.

Clinical features include marked tachypnoea, dry cough and fever. Hypoxia is often marked and precedes radiological change. The typical X-ray shows diffuse, bilateral alveolar disease originating at the hilum and progressing peripherally.

For a definitive diagnosis *P. carinii* must be identified in lung tissue by fibreoptic bronchoscopy or open lung biopsy. Treatment is with either i) Trimethoprim-sulphamethoxazole (co-trimoxazole) or ii) pentamidine isethionate. Untreated, the fatality rate approaches 100%, but is reduced to 25% with one of these agents. Up to 15% of patients who recover will have a second episode. Chemoprophylaxis for high-risk patients is with co-trimoxazole which is dependable for only as long as the drug is taken.

9 a) A Meckel's diverticulum presenting with haemorrhage. The differential diagnosis includes Peutz–Jeghers syndrome, hereditary haemorrhagic telangiectasia, Crohn's disease and Familial Polyposis Coli, but the normal appearance of perioral and perianal skin, oral mucosa and rectal mucosa make them unlikely candidates.

A Meckel's diverticulum represents the remains of the vitello-intestinal tract. It occurs in 2% of the population and is approximately 2 cm in length and situated 2 ft from the ileocaecal valve attached to the antimesenteric border. Heterotropic gastric mucosa and pancreatic tissue are occasionally found in the diverticulum.

The majority of patients are asymptomatic but recognized complications include: inflammation – symptoms and signs mimic appendicitis, intestinal obstruction and haemorrhage. Bleeding occurs from adjacent small intestine mucosa when ectopic gastric mucosa is present, and an acute bleed usually manifests as the passage of bright red rectal blood. Alternatively low grade blood loss may occur and complicate chronic peptic ulceration. Clinically any child with painless rectal bleeding should be assumed to have a Meckel's diverticulum.

b) Arteriography is of value in defining the site of bleeding when blood loss exceeds 1 ml/min. Alternatively abdominal scanning following injection of isotope labelled red blood cells may help in localizing the site of blood loss.

99 m-technetium scanning has a role in outlining ectopic gastric mucosa as the isotope is concentrated in gastric mucosa. Laparotomy is often necessary not only to confirm the diagnosis, but also to provide definitive treatment.

10 a) Hypergastrinaemia resulting in recurrent peptic ulceration. Up to 80% of patients develop a varying degree of steatorrhoea following partial gastrectomy.

The fall in serum gastrin levels during the secretin test in a patient who has undergone a Polya gastrectomy is highly suggestive of **retained gastric antrum**. In contrast the gastrin level in cases of a gastrin-secreting tumour (Zollinger–Ellison syndrome) rise during the secretin test. In normal individuals gastrin levels fall during the test.

b) The diagnosis of retained gastric antrum should be confirmed at laparotomy.

11 a) **Chronic hepatitis B-induced hepatitis,** possibly acquired during childhood. The factors which determine whether a hepatitis B infection becomes chronic or full recovery occurs are not known. Ten percent of patients after an acute infection develop one of three chronic syndromes: i) normal histology but a chronic carrier; ii) chronic persistent hepatitis; iii) chronic active hepatitis which may progress to cirrhosis and is an important risk for the development of primary hepatocellular carcinoma. During the first years of chronic infection, virus replication is high; patients are HBs Ag and HBe Ag-positive but are e antibody-negative and are highly infectious. Later, patients develop antibodies to first HBc Ag then HBe Ag and finally HBs Ag. After many years HBs Ag and HBe Ag may be undetectable, although antibodies to the core protein (HBc Ag) remain detectable.

b) Investigations: i) HBe Ag, HBc antibody and Hbs antibody to assess the patient's infectivity and immune response to the virus; ii) a liver biopsy and liver ultrasound to assess hepatic damage and any continuing liver inflammation or cirrhosis.

c) Indications for therapy include i) infectivity, e.g. HBe Ag-positive patients, and ii) evidence of progressive liver disease (chronic active hepatitis). Decompensated cirrhosis is a contraindication. Treatment with antiviral agents and possibly interferon is useful even if the virus has become integrated into the host genome; improvement of the inflammatory liver disease will occur if viral replication is inhibited.

12 a) This man has spinal cord compression with nerve root involvement resulting in a sensory level at T10 and evidence of both pyramidical weakness and dorsal column involvement. Rectal tone is often preserved until late in spinal cord compression.

Radiology shows destruction of T8 and T9 vertebrae. The main differential diagnosis is between a malignant and an infectious process. Involvement of two adjacent vertebrae and loss of the disc space strongly suggests infection rather than malignancy. Night sweats which resolved after antibiotic therapy are a further clue. The lack of an acute phase response and normal white blood count do not favour malignancy. Spinal osteomyelitis may be associated with little systemic upset and furthermore he had received antibiotics. The change in bowel habit is solely the result of opiate analgesia.

Note: Back pain which radiates in a dermatomal distribution suggests nerve root involvement and therefore a disease process which involves the epidural space. The radiological appearance may lag behind the clinical disease by weeks or months.

b) CT scanning or MRI scanning. Isotope bone scans are helpful only when the plain X-rays are normal.

The treatment of spinal compression is urgent decompression, and the prognosis is related to the speed of diagnosis as decompression, to be successful, must be undertaken early. There are two mechanisms causing neurological damage:
i) the formation of an epidural abscess with a mass effect, and
ii) thrombosis of the spinal arteries.

The treatment of spinal osteomyelitis is intravenous antibiotics for 6 weeks. Accurate microbiological diagnosis is essential and may be obtained by guided biopsy, if surgery is not required for spinal decompression.

The main organisms implicated in spinal osteomyelitis are *Staphylococcus aureus* (60%), enterobacteriae (30%), acid-fast bacillae, brucella, *Haemophilus influenzae*, nocardia, candida, and *Treponema pallidum*. Organisms usually spread via the blood stream but direct invasion may occur, e.g. from a pharyngeal abscess.

13 a) Bartter's syndrome. The patient is normotensive and investigations show a hypochloraemic hypokalaemic alkalosis together with high urine potassium loss.

Bartter's syndrome is characterized by severe renal potassium wasting and an inability to concentrate the urine. Histologically, hyperplasia of the juxtaglomerular apparatus is seen.

The syndrome usually presents in childhood and an increased familial incidence has been noted. Children present with weakness, vomiting, polyuria, nocturnal enuresis, growth retardation and low IQ.

The diagnosis depends on demonstration of renal potassium loss in the presence of a hypokalaemic metabolic alkalosis, elevated aldosterone secretion and increased plasma renin activity, in a normotensive individual.

Abnormal potassium loss in the urine is suggested by the finding of more than 20 mmol of potassium in the urine per 24 hours with a plasma potassium of less than 3 mmol/l. Treatment consists of potassium supplementation with or without one aldosterone antagonist. Non-steroidal anti-inflammatory agents which interfere with tubular prostaglandin production have been shown to correct the hypokalaemic alkalosis and hyper-reninism. Some patients have hypomagnesaemia and require magnesium supplements.

The differential diagnosis of a metabolic hypokalaemic alkalosis includes:

1) Adrenal tumours^
2) Elevated ACTH levels
3) Diuretic abuse
4) Villous adenoma*
5) Laxative abuse*

^ Blood pressure usually high
* Are associated with diarrhoea and the urine potassium excretion is low

14 a) The neuroleptic malignant syndrome is a well-recognized idiosyncratic side-effect of antidopaminergic drugs such as phenothiazines and butyrophenones which are used in the management of schizophrenia. The syndrome usually develops insidiously soon after treatment is initiated, and is characterized by hyperthermia, tachycardia, muscle rigidity, dysphagia and impaired consciousness. Creatinine kinase levels are elevated and reflect muscle damage. Death from respiratory failure is not uncommon; other complications include renal failure due to myoglobinuria, metabolic acidosis and cardiac failure. The increased muscle tone appears to be presynaptically mediated and recovery occurs when neuroleptic serum levels fall.

Management of the syndrome includes active cooling, rehydration and correction of metabolic acidosis, and ventilation when necessary. Intravenous dantrolene, which inhibits calcium efflux from muscle, and dopamine antagonists e.g. bromocriptine, have been used with varying effect to reduce muscle tone.

15 a) A hypochloraemic hypokalaemic metabolic alkalosis.

b) Pyloric stenosis.

c) The patient's urine may be inappropriately acidic.

d) In pyloric stenosis, vomiting of HCl stomach contents occurs (no communication between stomach and duodenum) H^+ and Cl^- are lost and HCO_{3-} is generated in the extracellular fluid resulting in a hypochloraemic alkalosis.

Urinary bicarbonate loss may be reduced in addition, due to: i) reduced GFR, and ii) a reduced chloride concentration in the glomerular filtrate, limiting resorption of sodium in the proximal tubule. More sodium is then available for exchange with H^+ and K^+, causing the urine to be inappropriately acid as H^+ secretion stimulates HCO_{3-} reabsorption. The fall in chloride may also increase the loss of potassium in exchange for sodium.

As a result of these changes, there is a *rise* in plasma bicarbonate, a *rise* in pH, with a *fall* in chloride. A low potassium results from a combination of gut loss (though this will be less marked than in normal vomiting), alkalosis (resulting in loss into cells), and increased urinary loss as explained above.

Answer to questions 16A–16B

16A a) Methyldopa-induced haemolytic anaemia.
b) Direct anti-human globulin test

16B a) De Quervain's thyroiditis (subacute thyroiditis). This occurs most commonly in young women. The exact aetiology is unknown, though a viral aetiology has been implicated. Often the initial presentation is of an upper respiratory tract infection with fever, sore throat and dysphagia. The thyroid gland is typically diffusely tender. Circulating thyroid hormone levels are high and signs of thyrotoxicosis may be present. Typically there is low or absent uptake of radioactive tracer on scanning.

b) The majority of cases respond to treatment with simple analgesics. Severe cases warrant a course of oral prednisolone. In the majority of cases the illness is short-lived and the patient is left euthyroid, but permanent hypothyroidism may result in some cases.

17 a) i) Metastatic malignancy with widespread meningeal and base-of-skull deposits.

   ii) Motor Neurone Disease (MND).

b) i) Metastatic malignancy is the more likely – ptosis and upper cranial nerve signs are rare in MND.

c) Electromyography will facilitate the diagnosis of MND. Skull X-ray, CT brain scan and an isotope bone scan may be required to demonstrate meningeal or base-of-skull tumour deposits. Malignant cells may be found on CSF examination.

Motor neurone disease is a disease characterized by selective degeneration of the motor neurones involving both the corticospinal pathways and those originating in the motor nuclei of the brainstem and anterior horn cells of the spinal cord. The aetiology is uncertain apart from several rare familial varieties. Trauma, toxins and viruses may all be involved in susceptible individuals. It is slightly more common in men, symptoms usually arising between 50 and 70 years of age. The symptoms are usually insidious and depend on the relative predominance of lower and upper motor neurone symptoms. There are three main clinical pictures:

Progressive muscular atrophy

Progressive bulbar palsy

Amyotrophic lateral sclerosis.

The diagnosis is based on clinical findings of upper and lower motor neurone signs in the absence of sensory signs. Histologically the grey matter of the anterior horns is small and the anterior roots are wasted. In view of the inevitably fatal and progressive nature of the disease it is important that the diagnosis is established, and this is based on EMG findings of spontaneous fibrillation on mechanical stimulation, duration and amplitude of action potentials greater than normal and a marked reduction in the number of spikes on maximal contraction due to the decreased number of motor units available for contraction. The rate of progression of the condition is highly variable: progressive bulbar palsy has the worst prognosis (mean survival 2 years) and pure progressive muscular atrophy the best (survival up to 8 years).

18 a) The most likely diagnosis is coeliac disease – the symptoms were present long before his holiday in Malaysia. The history is entirely compatible with malabsorption. The proximal muscle weakness may be attributed to osteomalacia subsequent to vitamin D malabsorption – corrected serum calcium is low, serum phosphate is low and alkaline phosphatase is high.

b) i) The diagnosis of coeliac disease is confirmed by jejunal biopsy. The initial biopsy classically shows subtotal villous atrophy which subsequently improves on a gluten-free diet. In adults it is not necessary to re-biopsy after a trial reintroduction of gluten.

ii) Measure serum levels of Vitamin B_{12}, folic acid, iron, TIBC and vitamin D.

c) The patient should be placed on a gluten-free diet. It may take up to 1 year for symptomatic improval to occur. Dietary supplements of Vitamin D, folic acid and iron should be given; these become unnecessary once the patient has responded to the gluten-free diet.

A differential diagnosis of the causes of subtotal villous atrophy includes:
1) Infectious enteritis in children
2) Giardiasis
3) Lymphoma
4) Whipple's disease
5) Hypogammaglobulinaemia
6) Cow's milk protein intolerance.

19 a) A is the interventricular septum. It is grossly thickened. Asymmetric septal hypertrophy is characteristic of hypertrophic obstructive cardiomyopathy. B is the closed mitral valve.

The anterior movement of the mitral valve during systole is a feature of hypertrophic obstructive cardiomyopathy.

b) During systole, ventricular ejection occurs and must traverse the space between mitral valve apparatus and septum (space C). In hypertrophic obstructive cardiomyopathy this is narrowed and causes functional outflow obstruction. With squatting, the peripheral vascular resistance increases, and the corresponding increase in systolic blood pressure causes dilatation of the aortic root. This reduces the functional obstruction by increasing the space at C.

c) Atrial and ventricular arrhythmias are a feature of hypertrophic obstructive cardiomyopathy and usually underlie syncope. There is controversy as to whether functional outflow obstruction is ever significant enough to lead to syncope.

20 a) The most likely diagnosis is Mycoplasma pneumoniae. The man presented with an atypical pneumonia associated with hepatitis, erythema multiforme and cold agglutinins and subsequently developed a myocarditis. Extrapulmonary manifestations of *M. pneumoniae* occur in over 10% of cases, generally within 3 weeks of the respiratory symptoms. The most important complications in terms of morbidity and mortality are cardiac (myocarditis and pericarditis) and neurological (meningitis, meningo-encephalitis, ascending paralysis, transverse myelitis, cranial nerve palsies, cerebellar ataxia and a poliomyelitis-like illness). The other extrapulmonary problems are more common, including skin rashes (25%), hepatitis, pancreatitis (rare), cold agglutinins (50%), haemolytic anaemia, bullous myringitis, thrombocytopenia, arthritis, and rarely, glomerulonephritis.

b) i) To confirm a diagnosis of *M. pneumoniae*: isolation of the organism from the respiratory system and mycoplasma serology. Culture is slow and not always available. A fourfold rise in antibody titre with a peak at 3–4 weeks suggests a recent infection. A rise in the cold agglutinin titre and the detection of specific IgM antibodies also suggest recent infection.

ii) Tests to exclude other atypical infections including legionnaire's disease, Q fever, psittacosis and viral infections (Coxsackie A and B and CMV)

Treatment of *Mycoplasma pneumoniae* is with erythromycin or tetracycline. Early treatment probably decreases the frequency of extrapulmonary complications, many of which are autoimmune in origin.

21 a) Gilbert's syndrome. The only abnormality is an elevated level of unconjugated bilirubin and the episode of jaundice was preceded by loss of appetite and reduced calorie intake.
Gilbert's syndrome encompasses a number of inherited metabolic abnormalities (presumed autosomal dominant in nature) which result in mildly elevated levels of unconjugated bilirubin. In many patients the primary defect is one of conjugation due to low levels of bilirubin uridine diphosphate glucoronate glucoronyl transferase. The elevated bilirubin level is usually insufficient to produce clinical jaundice. The diagnosis is usually made when calorie intake is reduced. This has the effect of raising the serum levels of unconjugated bilirubin in the absence of haemolysis. On reducing calorie intake to less than 400 calories, unconjugated bilirubin levels double in normal patients and also those with Gilbert's disease. In the latter group, due to the higher starting value, clinical jaundice is often apparent.
A nicotinic acid provocation test may also be used to aid diagnosis. Intravenous nicotinic acid elevates the level of unconjugated bilirubin by at least 17 μmol/l and there is delayed clearance compared to normal controls.
Liver biopsy is not essential for diagnosis; the histology is usually unremarkable but may show an increase in centrilobular lipofuscin. The long term prognosis is excellent.

22 a) Rhabdomyolysis (with myoglobinuria)
   b) Three possible reasons:
      i) status epilepticus
      ii) alcohol excess – note the low red cell transketolase level and elevated gamma glutamyl transpeptidase
      iii) a prolonged period of unconsciousness.
Rhabdomyolysis may also occur with sepsis, trauma, after prolonged exertion and following burns and electrocution. Biochemically it is characterized by a massively disproportionate rise in serum creatinine from muscle damage compared with blood urea, hyperkalaemia, increased muscle enzymes (AST and CPK), hypocalcaemia as a consequence of calcium binding to damaged muscle, and hyperuricaemia. Myoglobin is detected in the urine and if in high enough concentration will turn the urine red-brown. Myoglobinuria gives a false positive dipstick result for blood but can be distinguished from haemoglobinuria by the ammonium sulphate test, which gives a coloured precipitate with haemoglobinuria and a coloured supernatant with myoglobinuria. Treatment is principally supportive, although alkalinization of the urine may ameliorate tubular damage and the development of acute tubular necrosis; the renal lesion will resolve spontaneously but a period of dialysis may be necessary. Non-symptomatic hypocalcaemia should not be treated as the calcium will deposit uselessly in the muscle.

23 a) **Lupus nephritis**
   b) Sub-endothelial and intramembranous deposits typical of membranous glomerulonephritis.
   c) The prognosis of nephritis in systemic lupus erythematosus is variable. Control of the patient's hypertension is important, and careful monitoring of renal function and protein excretion is necessary. Aggressive immunosuppressive therapy may be required.
   There are 3 diseases in which linear IgG deposition may be reported on the glomerular basement membrane: i) anti-GBM disease (Goodpasture's syndrome), ii) diabetes mellitus, and iii) systemic lupus erythematosus. Goodpasture's syndrome is unlikely with this degree of hypertension and nephrotic range proteinuria, and diabetes mellitus is also unlikely with a normal glycosylated Hb level.
   Lupus nephritis is now classified according to the histological features:

   Class I – normal
   Class IIa – electron microscopic or immunofluorescent evidence of mesangial disease
   Class IIb – mesangial hypercellularity
   Class III – focal segmental glomerulonephritis (<50% of glomeruli involved)
   Class IV – diffuse glomerulonephritis (>50% of glomeruli involved)
   Type V – membranous nephropathy.

Refractory hypertension is common in lupus nephritis and an important pitfall in its diagnosis is the apparently innocuous urinary sediment underlying an aggressive nephritis.

24 a) **The glucose profile shows a lag storage pattern.** The 30-minute sample is high and exceeds the renal threshold for glucose (usually 10 mmol/l) resulting in detectable glycosuria. This profile implies a delay in the hepatic storage of glucose. The initial high blood glucose levels lead to an increased insulin secretion which results in the subsequent hypoglycaemia.
   b) The lag storage pattern may occur in apparently normal individuals but is a well-recognized complication of gastrectomy or gastrojejunostomy when rapid absorption of blood glucose occurs.
   Other causes of a lag storage curve include severe liver disease associated with decreased glycogenolysis, and thyrotoxicosis.
   Note: causes of a flat glucose tolerance curve where levels fail to rise normally following an oral glucose load include:
   1) Normal individuals
   2) Malabsorption states
   3) Addison's disease
   4) Hypopituitarism (with growth hormone deficiency).

25 a) This patient has had symptoms of malaise for 7 months, has several spider naevi and a biochemical hepatitis. The most likely diagnosis in this case is an autoimmune chronic active hepatitis. Vitiligo, the positive ANA and raised immunoglobulins all suggest an autoimmune aetiology.

The differential diagnosis of chronic hepatitis includes:

1) Autoimmune hepatitis (often associated with other autoimmune diseases).
2) Chronic viral hepatitis serological tests available for Hepatitis B, Hepatitis C and Hepatitis D.
3) Alcohol.
4) Drugs, e.g. methyldopa, nitrofurantoin, and isoniazid.
5) Wilson's disease.
6) α_1 anti-trypsine deficiency.

Occasionally early primary biliary cirrhosis and primary sclerosing cholangitis may present with a biochemical hepatitis and be confused with chronic active hepatitis.

b) Appropriate investigations include a liver biopsy, organ-specific and non-organ specific autoantibodies, anti-hepatitis C antibodies and serum caeruloplasmine and urinary copper estimation.

c) Immediate management would include stopping the contraceptive pill and alcohol, which may be contributing to the liver damage. Immunosuppression with corticosteroids forms the mainstay of treatment; azathioprine may be added as a steroid sparing agent.

Autoimmune chronic active hepatitis is commoner in women than in men and presents in two peaks between 10 and 25 years of age and between 50 and 65 years of age. In addition to a biochemical hepatitis characterized by a raised aspartate amino-transferase level with a normal or only slightly elevated alkaline phosphatase, and the stigmata of chronic liver disease, 50% have other systemic symptoms including fever, arthralgia, vasculitic skin lesions, haemolytic anaemia, thrombocytopenia and leucopenia. A number of patients have other autoimmune diseases such as systemic lupus erythematosus, fibrosing alveolitis, diabetes mellitus, autoimmune thyroid disease, kerato conjunctivitis sicca and ulcerative colitis. Typically patients have a positive ANA, raised immunoglobulins, primarily IgG, and a high titre of anti-smooth muscle antibodies. Recently antibodies against liver membrane and mitochondrial components (different to those found in primary biliary cirrhosis) have been detected, which appear to be specific for autoimmune chronic active hepatitis.

Liver histology shows inflammation in the portal and periportal areas with 'piecemeal' necrosis. In advanced disease liver architecture is disrupted and healing with fibrosis eventually leads to a macronodular cirrhosis.

26 a) Digoxin, verapamil and adenosine cause AV nodal block and will increase the degree in this case or even cause complete AV dissociation.
Isoprenaline, atropine and imipramine will increase conduction through the node and might relieve the 2:1 block demonstrated.

27 a) Pregnancy.
During pregnancy the elevated levels of oestrogens and progesterone result in a number of metabolic changes which include:
1) A reduction in total plasma proteins and albumin.
2) An increase in several binding proteins including thyroid binding globulin (therefore increased bound T4 and total T4 but normal free T4), cortisol binding globulin and transferrin. In each case the 'total' bound substance is increased but the free unbound is normal.
Note: any cause of high oestrogens, e.g. the contraceptive pill or treatment with stilboestrol will produce a similar effect.
3) Elevated serum cholesterol levels.
4) Glycosuria.
5) Late in pregnancy there may be lactosuria which will give a positive Clinitest but negative Clinistix.
6) In the last trimester of pregnancy, levels of alkaline phosphatase are usually elevated because of increased heat-stable alkaline phosphatase from the placenta.
7) Immediately following labour, several enzymes including aspartate transaminase, alkaline phosphatase and creatinine phosphokinase are elevated.

28 a) i) **Anorexia nervosa** – the most common reason for weight loss in this age group.

ii) **Brucellosis** – she may have been drinking unpasteurized milk in Greece.

iii) **A second malignancy** – Hodgkin's disease is most likely with a history of fevers, and 10 years is an appropriate time interval.

b) i) Admit for observation of eating pattern.

ii) Brucella antibody levels; IgG and IgM in acute infection, IgG and IgA in chronic infection.

The diagnosis of anorexia nervosa is a clinical one, based on the following findings: considerable weight loss, specific psychopathology associated with guilt about eating, loss of control and a disturbed body image where the patient perceives herself as fat. Patients diet excessively, exercise keenly and may have experienced a recent emotional upset. On examination the patient may have signs of extreme weight loss, blue-cold hands and feet, dry skin with downly hair over the nape of neck, cheeks, forearms and legs, and a low pulse pressure is often observed. LH, FSH and oestradiol levels are abnormally low. In the male, plasma LH and testosterone levels are low and there is loss of sexual interest and potency. Other blood results are likely to be normal unless self-induced vomiting is associated with electrolyte abnormalities. The increased incidence in Western society and among higher social classes, suggest that the aetiology is related to culturally determined attitudes. The aims of treatment are to obtain the patient's confidence and a degree of cooperation, restore their weight to a healthy level, reduce residual disability and shorten the duration of the illness.

Brucellosis is a zoonosis caused by *Brucella melitensis, B. suis* or *B. abortus*, in decreasing order of frequency in man. The organism is a small Gram-negative coccobacillus which is an intracellular pathogen. Primary infection may be acute, chronic or subclinical. It may be contracted from milk or soft cheeses, tending animals and handling the carcasses of infected animals and is an occupational disease of farmers and related professions. The bacillus enters across mucous membranes, is phagocytosed, reaches lymph nodes and there replicates. It is released when the cell is disrupted and reaches the liver and spleen.

Chills, sweats, aches and pains, general lethargy and episodic fevers are typical. Granulocytopenia may be the first clue to the diagnosis and lymphocytosis can occur when it is chronic. The diagnosis is made either serologically or by isolation of the organism from blood cultures, bone marrow aspirate, or pus.

Treatment is with tetracycline if the condition is diagnosed early, otherwise streptomycin must be added. Doxycycline and rifampicin are also an effective therapeutic combination. Spontaneous resolution occurs after months without treatment; relapse is common and may occur within 2 months of treatment.

29 a) The most likely diagnosis is **falciparum malaria** with acute tubular necrosis. The features suggesting malaria are:

1) An intermittent fever not responding to antibiotics, with a history of travel to a malaria area. The incubation period is normally 8–25 days; however, partial antimalaria prophylaxis and the non-specific features often result in considerable delay in presentation.
2) Frontal headaches, non-productive cough, myalgias and diffuse abdominal pains are typical of *Plasmodium falciparum*, chest pains and arthralgias are also recognized features. Malaria in the early stages may easily be confused with a viral illness.
3) Personality changes are the earliest signs of cerebral malaria. The lack of focal neurology, both on examination and on CT-scan, and the normal CSF findings make other diagnoses less likely.
4) The severity of the normochromic normocytic anaemia suggests malaria rather than another infection. Both haemolysis and dyserythropoiesis contribute to the anaemia in malaria. Massive haemolysis leads to haemoglobinuria 'blackwater' fever.
5) Renal failure. Acute tubular necrosis is the main cause of acute renal failure in falciparum malaria. Several mechanisms contribute: i) intravascular haemolysis and haemoglobinuria, ii) hypovolaemia and renal vasoconstriction, and iii) blockage of small blood vessels. *Plasmodium malariae* and *Plasmodium falciparum* may cause a nephrotic syndrome, with evidence of immune complex deposition in the mesangium and glomerular basement membrane. A unique feature of falciparum malaria is that parasitized RBC have an increased ability to stick to endothelium; this is related to protuberances on the RBC surface expressing a molecule similar to thrombospondin which binds to fibronectin. Sequestration and blockage of parasitized RBC in capillaries of brain and kidney play an important role in damage to these organs.

b) Thick and thin blood films should be obtained to identify RBC parasites.

The differential diagnosis is obviously wide and includes other infections such as infective endocarditis and brucellosis. Syphilis, visceral Leishmaniasis, ascending cholangitis and AIDS are all very unlikely; the lack of lymph nodes or hepatosplenomegaly makes neoplasia (such as Hodgkin's disease) or sarcoidosis unlikely.

c) Treatment – cautious rehydration, intravenous quinine is given for 7 days followed by a single dose of pyrimethamine-sulfadoxine (Fansidar). Quinine levels should be measured to monitor therapy.

Note: Classical tertian or subtertian fever strikes are rarely seen in falciparum malaria.

30 a) The most likely diagnosis is Farmer's lung, an extrinsic allergic alveolitis, in which the patient is hypersensitive to spores of thermophyllic actiomycetes in mouldy hay. Extrinsic allergic alveolitis refers to a group of conditions in which inhaled organic dusts trigger a hypersensitivity reaction, including Farmer's lung, Bird-fancier's lung, Mushroom-worker's lung, etc. Although many of these conditions are associated with specific precipitins (antibodies to the presumed antigen) complement activation by immune complexes (type III hypersensitivity) is no longer thought to be the only or even the most important mechanism causing lung damage. Cell-mediated (type IV) hypersensitivity is probably the most important process. Histology shows extensive lymphocyte infiltration of the alveolar walls and in more advanced cases granuloma formation and lung fibrosis. The acute form presents as an influenza-like illness (malaise, myalgia, fever, headache) and breathlessness with a dry cough but no wheeze. The symptoms commence 3–9 hours after exposure to the sensitizing antigen. A period of exposure (several weeks to months) is required before the first attacks are noticed. In severe forms hypoxia may be profound and the chest X-ray shows a ground glass appearance. In the chronic form the symptoms are less dramatic and there is gradual onset of dyspnoea on exertion. The most consistent physical sign is fine crepitations heard throughout the lung. Patients may present with lung fibrosis or cor pulmonale which may be difficult to distinguish from cryptogenic fibrosing alveolitis or sarcoid. The fibrosis may be predominantly in the upper lobes and simulate the chest X-ray changes of tuberculosis.

b) The most important step is to take an occupational history to identify the causative antigen and confirm appropriate exposure. Further investigations should include a lung biopsy, bronchoalveolar lavage and examination of the serum for precipitating antibodies.

Investigation of extrinsic allergic alveolitis involves pulmonary assessment, antigen identification and history of relevant exposure, and finally immunological confirmation of the hypersensitivity. Lung function tests show a restrictive ventilatory defect with some air trapping and occasionally some evidence of large airways obstruction. Biopsy is the most sensitive way of distinguishing between cryptogenic fibrosing alveolitis, other granulomatous disease and extrinsic allergic alveolitis. Bronchoalveolar lavage findings are similar to sarcoid – with increased lymphocytes, unlike cryptogenic fibrosing alveolitis, where polymorphs predominate. The finding of precipitating IgG antibodies is not diagnostic since such antibodies are found in healthy people who have had appropriate exposure. If the diagnosis remains doubtful then challenge tests using inhaled antigen may be considered.

Treatment is avoidance of the responsible antigen. Steroids may be useful in a severe acute extrinsic allergic alveolitis. Patients are eligible for compensation under the Industrial Injuries Acts.

31 A
  a) Autosomal dominant with inheritance.

  B
  a) From the family tree males are affected and unaffected females are able to transmit the trait. Therefore the likely mode of transmission is X-linked recessive.

  b) The risk to A and his children is zero as A will receive a Y chromosome from his affected father. We can assume the chance that a new mutation which would give rise to the same condition can be ignored. In the case of patient B, his great-grandfather was affected, implying that his grandmother was a carrier and therefore the probability that his mother was a carrier is 1/2; his risk is therefore 1/4. The mother of patient C has an affected brother, therefore the probability that she is a carrier is 1/2; the chance that her daughter will also be a carrier is 1/4.

  c) The principal X-linked recessive conditions encountered are Haemophilia A and B, Duchenne and Becker's muscular dystrophy, glucose-6-dehydrogenase deficiency, nephrogenic diabetes insipidus, Hunter's syndrome, Lesch–Nyhan syndrome, colour blindness and Fabry's disease.

32 a) Post-infectious malabsorption syndrome (formerly called tropical sprue). Post-infectious malabsorption syndrome may be defined as a chronic malabsorption syndrome (greater than 2 months' duration) in which an abnormal bacterial flora – typically mixed aerobic enterobacteriae – is present in the small intestine.

The disease is common in India, the Indian subcontinent, the West Indies and South America but less common in Africa, and occurs not only in travellers but also in the indigenous population.

The disease usually starts after several years' residence in the tropics, with an acute attack of diarrhoea believed to be infective in origin. This is followed by colonization of the small intestine with a mixed population of aerobic enterobacteriae. Histologically there is evidence of mucosal damage though villous atrophy is not a feature. Severe folic acid depletion is usually present by 4 months and exacerbates the mucosal damage. Plasma levels of enteroglucagon are high, which serves to reduce intestinal motility, encouraging the persistence of an abnormal flora.

Following the acute attack of diarrhoea which may be bloody, diarrhoea becomes chronic, with bulky stool, and colicky abdominal pain is common. Symptoms and signs are those of malabsorption and vitamin deficiencies. Fever, weight loss, pigmentation and glossitis are common. Folic acid deficiency is often severe and B_{12} deficiency may occur as in this case, resulting in doral column loss and loss of ankle jerks. Osteomalacia leads to proximal weakness.

The diagnosis may only be made when all other causes, especially infections with giardia and strongyloides, have been ruled out.

b) The differential diagnosis includes:
1) Coeliac disease
2) Crohn's disease
3) Infections:
   Giardia lamblia
   Strongyloides stercoralis
   Cryptosporidium
4) Small intestine lymphoma
5) Kwashiorkor
6) Ileocaecal tuberculosis
7) Hypolactasia

c) Treatment regimen: a combination of tetracycline with folic acid supplementation usually results in rapid clinical improvement.

33 a) Lumbar spinal stenosis and claudication of the cauda equina.

b) Myelography with or without CT-scanning is the investigation of choice. Surgery is the definitive treatment.

There are a number of mechanisms which may lead to stenosis of the lumbar canal, including osteoarthritis with hypertrophy of the facet joints, disc prolapse, surgery, spondylolisthesis, Paget's disease, neoplasia and infection. Any of these conditions may be superimposed on a congenitally narrow spinal canal.

Typically the symptoms develop slowly and may be very vague. Back pain as such is not a feature. The neurological symptoms often do not fit into any clear root or peripheral nerve distribution. In chronic cases there may be quadriceps wasting. The A-P diameter of the lumbar spinal canal is narrowed during extension, which appears to interfere with the blood supply to the cord; by stooping forward the A-P diameter is increased, so rapidly relieving the symptoms.

Normal plain radiographs of the spine do not exclude the diagnosis. Intermittent claudication may easily be distinguished from this syndrome by Doppler examination of the pulses before and after exercise.

34 a) End diastolic diameter exceeds 5.5 cm and there is therefore left ventricular dilatation.

b) Any space behind the posterior wall of the left ventricle is abnormal; it represents a pericardial effusion.

c) i) A paradoxical rise in the jugular venous pressure on inspiration – 'Kussmaul's sign'.

   ii) Pulsus paradoxus – an exaggerated fall in the systolic blood pressure on inspiration (normally less than 10 mmHg).

These signs only occur if there is significant haemodynamic compromise as a result of the effusion.

35 a) Gonococcal arthritis.

b) Investigations aim to isolate the organism (Gram-negative intracellular diplococci) from the urethra, vagina, throat, synovial fluid, blood, or from a pustule. Gonococci are notoriously difficult to grow in culture; blood cultures will be positive in less than 20% and synovial cultures in less than 50%.
Neisseria gonococci are a frequent cause of septic arthritis in young people. Radiology of the joint is normal unless the condition is left untreated, when severe destruction can take place.

Gonorrhea occurs in females as frequently as in males, however, affected females generally have fewer symptoms and may act as asymptomatic carriers. Pregnant and menstruating females are more prone to haematogenous spread from vaginal foci. Arthritis and a vesiculopustular skin rash are the commonest complications. Others include endocarditis, meningitis, myocarditis, and hepatitis. A mild fever and leucocytosis, raised ESR and CRP accompany gonococcaemia. Tenosynovitis, particularly of the wrists, hands, feet or Achilles tendon, occurs in two-thirds of cases. Tenosynovitis, a fever and one or two swollen joints in a young person strongly suggest the diagnosis.

36 a) The clinical picture of an acute illness characterized by fever, a widespread rash, diarrhoea, myalgia, drowsiness and hypotension is typical of the **toxic shock syndrome**. The toxic shock syndrome, due to a toxin-producing staphylococcus, is usually associated with tampon use in menstruating females but can also occur in association with staphylococcal conjunctivitis, pharyngitis, infected burns and local abscesses.

Definitive criteria for the diagnosis include:

1) A temperature >39°C.
2) A widespread erythematous macular rash.
3) Hypotension systolic pressure <90 mmHg or a postural diastolic drop.
4) Toxic action on at least 3 systems, e.g. diarrhoea or vomiting, raised creatinine phosphokinase or myalgia, raised urea and creatinine, thrombocytopenia <100 × 10⁹/l, drowsiness and confusion.

A local source of infection – eyes, oropharynx, vagina etc.

b) A vaginal examination should be performed and any tampon removed. The toxin-producing staphylococcus should be isolated from the primary site and/or the blood. Other infections such as streptococcal septicaemia, leptospirosis, measles and rickettsial infections must be excluded. A low threshold for examination of the cerebrospinal fluid should pertain if drowsiness is prominent.

c) Tampon removal prevents further absorption of toxin; parenteral flucloxacillin should be given initially and the specific sensitivity of the organism awaited. Shock should be treated with intravenous fluids and inotropic agents may be necessary.

37A a) Lithium toxicity would account for the drowsiness, tremor, thyroid function abnormalities and ECG changes. Hypernatraemia complicates lithium-induced nephrogenic diabetes insipidus, when the patient's conscious level prevents an adequate fluid intake necessary to compensate for the polyuria.

Lithium is primarily used in the treatment of manic depressive illness. Lithium is excreted by the kidneys and has a low therapeutic index. Regular drug monitoring is recommended at monthly intervals.

Theraputic levels of lithium – 0.4–1.2 mmol/l; toxicity occurs with levels >1.5 mmol/l and coma may occur with levels >2.5 mmol/l.

Recognized side effects of lithium include fine tremor, nausea and diarrhoea, low T4 and compensatory rise in TSH. Hypothyroidism may be apparent; polyuria and polydypsia are common and a few patients develop frank diabetes insipidus (lithium antagonizes the effect of ADH on the distal convoluted tubule and collecting ducts). Lithium may also induce a state of partial renal tubular acidosis. Symptoms of lithium toxicity include drowsiness, coarse tremor, vomiting, coma, fits, renal failure and cardiovascular collapse.

Lithium toxicity may be provoked by sodium depletion. Eighty percent of lithium filtered by the glomerulus is reabsorbed by the proximal convoluted tubule and this percentage is increased in sodium-depleted states

37B a) Hepatic encephalopathy due to alcoholic liver disease.

b) Hyponatraemia – secondary hyperaldosteronism.
Low urea – reduced hepatic synthesis.
Thrombocytopaenia – hypersplenism.
Macrocytosis and increased triglyceride levels are commonly found in alcoholic patients.

38 a) The diagnosis is progressive systemic sclerosis. Raynaud's phenomenon, pruritus, prolonged tanning and skin oedema are common features of early progressive systemic sclerosis. As the disease progresses major organs become involved, particularly the lungs, kidneys, gut and heart.

b) Complications:

1) Interstitial pneumonitis – she has shortness of breath on exertion, basal crackles and pulmonary function tests consistent with lung restriction (loss of lung volume and a reduced TLCO). Pulmonary manifestations, including interstitial pneumonitis, pulmonary fibrosis, pleural thickening and pleural effusions, are common in progressive systemic sclerosis and may occur early. Progressive interstitial lung disease may be complicated by pulmonary hypertension and right-sided heart failure, a frequent cause of death in progressive systemic sclerosis. Pulmonary hypertension secondary to an extensive pulmonary artery sclerosis may occur in the absence of pulmonary fibrosis. Treatment of interstitial pneumonitis and progressive lung fibrosis is immunosuppression with prednisolone and cytotoxic agents such as cyclophosphamide. A rare pulmonary complication of progressive systemic sclerosis is alveolar cell or bronchiolar carcinoma.

2) Renovascular hypertension – her blood pressure and her plasma creatinine levels are elevated (taking into consideration her age and urea level). Renovascular hypertension is generally a late but ominous complication of progressive systemic sclerosis, often leading to rapidly-progressive and irreversible renal failure. The onset of the hypertension is often sudden and may be heralded by headaches. Urgent control of the blood pressure as an inpatient is indicated. Often, even with control of the blood pressure, renal function continues to decline. Patients on corticosteroids appear to be more likely to present with malignant hypertension.

39 a) Hypogammaglobulinaemia with immunodeficiency. The clues are: chronic childhood infections (mostly bacterial), chronic diarrhoea which responds to antibiotics including metronidazole (*Giardia lamblia*), a chronic non-erosive arthritis and low immunoglobulins (normal albumin but a low total protein). An important differential diagnosis to consider is cystic fibrosis, but the low immunoglobulin level makes this unlikely.

b) Immunoglobulin levels, including subclasses.

c) Sandoglobulin (pooled human immunoglobulin) intravenously 2–4-weekly and penicillin V 500 mg daily.

The primary defect is unknown. Patients have normal numbers of B-cells and generally normal T-cell populations. There appears to be a defect in antibody production or secretion. Infections with pyogenic bacteria (particularly haemophilus, staphylococcus, streptococcus, and pseudomonas) and protozoa (*Giardia lamblia*) are the main clinical consequences of antibody deficiency. The majority of patients present in the second or third decade but any age is possible. (note: they do not present before 3–6 months of age as maternal antibodies provide protection). Lymphadenopathy is a common finding and typically histology shows granulomas.

Chronic respiratory tract infections may lead to brochiectasis, pulmonary fibrosis, cor pulmonale and early death.

The polyarthritis/arthralgia associated with hypogammaglobulinaemia is a symmetrical non-erosive polyarthritis which generally spares the hands and feet. Tenosynovitis can be prominent; rarely, rheumatoid nodules are seen. Synovial histology shows a mononuclear cell infiltrate but not the lymphoid hyperplasia seen in rheumatoid arthritis. Rheumatoid factors are absent. It is always important to consider the possibility of septic arthritis (particularly mycoplasma) in these patients.

Chronic diarrhoea is a common feature and is often due to chronic giardia infection; similarly patients with selective IgA deficiency also have this complication.

B_{12} deficiency and atrophic gastritis occur, without the antibodies associated with pernicious anaemia.

There is an increased incidence of autoimmune disease and malignancy. The possibility of a lymphoma must be considered if lymphadenopathy is a major feature. B_{12} deficiency and atrophic gastritis are not uncommonly seen in these patients.

40 a) Disseminated intravascular coagulation complicating acute promyelocytic leukaemia. The coagulation tests are diagnostic of disseminated intravascular coagulation a well-recognized complication of acute promyelocytic leukaemia. The characteristic coagulation abnormalities are thrombocytopenia (this may also be caused by infiltration of the marrow with blasts), prolongation of the prothrombin, partial thromboplastin and thrombin times, hypofibrinogenaemia and raised levels of fibrin degradation products.

b) The diagnosis of acute myeloid leukaemia can be confirmed by bone marrow examination which will reveal the characteristic hypergranular blasts. The granules contain a procoagulant which triggers disseminated intravascular coagulation, which may be the presenting feature of this type of leukaemia. Lysis of the blasts during chemotherapy may worsen the disseminated intravascular coagulation and treatment must include meticulous monitoring of coagulation and appropriate support with platelets and fresh frozen plasma. The role of heparin is controversial. Once in remission, acute promyelocytic leukaemia has one of the most favourable prognoses of AML.

Recognized causes of acute disseminated intravascular coagulation include:

1) Infections and toxins
   Gram-negative septicaemia, malaria, snake bite
2) Malignancy
   Disseminated malignancy, acute promyelocytic leukaemia
3) Obstetric causes
   Amniotic fluid embolism, abruptio placenta, retained fetus, eclampsia, antepartum haemorrhage
4) Miscellaneous
   Mismatched transfusion, major trauma, aortic dissection.

41 A a) Measurement of lung volumes TLC/RV to assess hyperinflation and air trapping. Bronchodilator response.

b) Emphysema

B a) Right pneumonectomy.

C a) Ventilatory failure.

b) Compensated respiratory acidosis.

42 a) Pyrexia; neck stiffness; focal neurological deficit; signs of ear or upper respiratory tract infection; papilloedema.

b) FBC, blood cultures, biochemical profile, blood glucose, head CT scan, lumbar puncture and CSF examination. There may be organisms visible on a Gram stain of the CSF, and neutrophils in the CSF, with a raised protein and low sugar. These findings indicate bacterial meningitis. A lymphocytosis suggests TB or more commonly, viral meningitis. Chemotherapy would be modified in the light of the microscopy and later culture results. The probable diagnosis is **meningococcal meningitis**.

c) Therapy with broad spectrum antibiotics usually intravenous benzyl penicillin and chloramphenicol (or new generation cephalosporins). Some neurological centres also recommend starting acyclovir particularly if there was any delay in obtaining the CSF results. Death; fits; residual neurological deficit; deafness; hydrocephalus; DIC; digital gangrene following vascular occlusion; circulatory collapse; Waterhouse – Friedrichsen syndrome; renal failure.

d) Immunoglobulins and serum complement estimation. Terminal pathway (C5–C9) complement deficiency predisposes particularly to meningococcal infection.

Typical CSF findings

	Pressure	Leucocytes	Protein	Glucose
Viral meningitis	Normal/ mild increase	50–500/mm 1⁰lymphocytes	0.4–1g/l	normal

Note: PMN may be increased during the first 24–48 hours.
CSF glucose levels may be low in cases of mumps or herpes meningitis.

	Pressure	Leucocytes	Protein	Glucose
Bacterial meningitis	Elevated	500–2000/mm³ 1° PMM	1–5g/l	Very low
Tuberculous meningitis	Elevated	50–500/mm³ 1° lymphocytes	1–5g/l	Usually low

Note: PMN may be increased during the first 24–48 hours.

	Pressure	Leucocytes	Protein	Glucose
Cryptococcal meningitis	Elevated	5–500/mm³ 1⁰lymphocytes	0.5–5g/l	Usually low
Carcinomatous meningitis (malignant cells often found)	N/elevated	5–300/mm³ 1⁰lymphocytes	0.5–5g/l	Normal/ reduced

43 a) Sexual history – he has just been to Bangkok; a history of urethritis.

b) Reiter's syndrome. Gonococcal infection.

c) The classic Reiter's triad consists of arthritis, conjunctivitis and urethritis. The seronegative arthritis typically affects the large and small joints of the lower limbs in an asymmetrical fashion; sacroileitis is common. Conjunctivitis and urethritis are usually mild.

Other recognized clinical features include plantar fasciitis, Achilles tendinitis, keratoderma blenorrhagica, circinate balanitis and painless buccal ulcers.

The initial disease is usually self-limiting but the arthritis becomes chronic in up to 60% of cases. Other late manifestations include uveitis, aortic regurgitation, conduction defects, pericarditis, pulmonary infiltrates, peripheral neuropathy and central nervous system involvement.

d) i) HLA-B27. Between 70–90% of patients with Reiter's syndrome are HLA-B27 positive.

  ii) Attacks may occur following intestinal infections, e.g. *Shigella flexneri* and *dysenteriae* (not sonnei), salmonella, yesinia and campylobacter.

44 a) The presence of polycythaemia with splenomegaly is highly suggestive of **primary proliferative polycythaemia** (polycythaemia rubra vera) a myeloproliferative disorder caused by the autonomous proliferation of a clone of erythroid cells which occurs in the absence of any erythropoietin drive. The diagnosis is supported by the elevated white cell and platelet counts and the raised serum urate (though in this case the patient's elevated uric acid level could be due to the thiazide diuretics or alcohol). There is no evidence of dehydration and blood gases are normal.

Polycythaemia refers to an increase in the haemoglobin concentration:

	Males	Females
Hb	>17.5g/dl	>15.5 g/dl
Red cell count	>6 × 10^{12}/l	>5.5 × 10^{12}/l
Haematocrit	>55%	>47%

Causes of polycythaemia may be subdivided into:
1) **Primary proliferative polycythaemia**
2) **Secondary causes**
   i) Inappropriate erythropoietin production, e.g. renal cysts, hypernephroma, cerebellar haemangioblastoma, hepatocellular carcinoma, uterine fibromas.
   ii) Compensatory increased erythropoietin production, e.g. high altitude, alveolar hypoventilation, cyanotic heart disease, smoking, methaemoglobinaemia.
3) **Relative polycythaemia**
Due to reduced plasma volume, e.g. dehydration, diuretics.

b) The first aim in the investigation of polycythaemia is to identify, caused by a true increase in red cell mass from relative polycythaemia, caused by a contraction of the plasma volume rather than any true increase in red cell mass. This may be achieved by isotopic measurement of red cell mass and plasma volume. Having established absolute polycythaemia, primary polycythaemia needs to be distinguished from the secondary causes.

Further appropriate investigations include:
1) Bone marrow examination – hypercellular with prominent megakaryocytes in primary proliferative polycythaemia and detection of erythropoietin-independent bone forming units.
2) Serum vitamin B_{12} binding capacity is high in primary proliferative polycythaemia.
3) Serum erythropoietin levels are normal or low in primary proliferative polycythaemia and high in other cases of secondary polycythaemia. In some patients further investigations to determine the source of inappropriately high erythropoietin levels will be necessary.

Treatment options for primary proliferative polycythaemia include venesection, cytotoxic drugs, e.g. chlorambucil and busulphan, and Phosphorus-32 therapy.

Answer to question 45

45 There is pulmonary hypertension with a right-to-left shunt. The most common cause is an **Eisenmenger ventricular septal defect**.

a) A right atrial pressure as high as this almost certainly suggests tricuspid regurgitation, secondary to right ventricular dilation and dysfunction. The waveform would be a dominant systolic wave, which is variously described as a: V-wave, S-wave or delta wave.

b) The low pulmonary artery diastolic pressure suggests pulmonary regurgitation. This often occurs as a result of prolonged pulmonary hypertension. There is no systolic gradient.

c) At 1 year the shunt would be left to right, and the pulmonary arterial tree is more prominent than usual in these circumstances ('pulmonary plethora'). With the onset of pulmonary hypertension of suprasystemic levels blood is diverted from right to left and away from the lungs giving oligaemia ('peripheral pruning') and the hilar pulmonary artery shadows become greatly enlarged.

Note: closure of the ventricular septal defect at this stage would lead to rapid death from right ventricular failure. With pulmonary vascular resistance of this magnitude the right ventricle is protected from fatal dilation and failure by the 'offloading' effect of the tricuspid incompetence and the systolic right-to-left shunt.

46 a) Adult Still's disease. The illness is characterized by arthritis, a macular rash, intermittent fever, splenomegaly, an elevated ESR and CRP, the anaemia of chronic disease, a neutrophil leucocytosis, mild hepatitis and a prompt and marked response to indomethacin.

Adult Still's disease is diagnosed on the basis of a triad of the typical rash, fever and arthritis, after excluding infection, other connective tissue disease, granulomatous diseases and neoplasia, and observing the often dramatic response to NSAIDS. The rash is non-puritic, maculopapular, a salmon pink colour, confined to the trunk and proximal limbs and associated with dermographism. It often comes and goes with the fever, which is high, spiking and often absent during the early part of the day.

The arthritis is typically an erosive oligoarthritis affecting large joints, particularly the wrists which may ankylose. Neck pain is also a feature.

Other features include marked constitutional symptoms, splenomegaly, lymphadenopathy, serositis, a normochromic normocytic anaemia and a marked acute phase response. The disease typically follows a relapsing course. Amyloidosis does not appear to be a risk, unlike in the childhood variety. Treatment is physiotherapy and non-steroidal anti-inflammatory agents. As has been emphasized the diagnosis is largely one of exclusion.

The differential diagnosis is wide and includes the following groups of diseases:

1) Infection e.g. viruses (including hepatitis B, parvovirus, rubella, adenovirus, cytomegalovirus, Epstein–Barr and human immunodeficency virus), infective endocarditis, rheumatic fever and Lyme disease.
2) Neoplasia, especially lymphomas.
3) Granulomatous disorders, sarcoidosis, Crohn's disease.
4) Connective tissue diseases.
5) Primary vasculitis syndromes, polyarteritis nodosa, giant-cell arteritis, etc.

The length of the history, anaemia of chronic disease and raised neutrophil count are against a virus infection. The patient has no risk factors for AIDS; the oral candida is more likely to be the result of having received antibiotics. Rheumatic fever is excluded since there is no evidence of a preceding streptococcal infection. Infective endocarditis caused by an unusual organism (e.g. coxiella or brucella) is possible but unlikely. Lyme disease is also unlikely; the rash and fever are atypical and the patient would be expected to respond to antibiotics.

There are no specific features suggesting granulomatous disease, vasculitis, or malignancy.

b) Further investigations should include serology to exclude coxiella, brucella, Lyme disease; an abdominal CT scan or ultrasound to exclude lymphadenopathy, and a liver and bone marrow biopsy to exclude granulomas. An atypical presentation of one of the connective tissue diseases is possible, despite the negative ANA; antibodies against specific nuclear and cytoplasmic antigens (ENAs) such as anti-Ro should be looked for.

47 a) The patient's fluid balance charts should be studied carefully. The precise anti-TB drugs he has been taking, and the duration of therapy should be ascertained.

b) Acute interstitial nephritis – Rifampicin is a likely cause. A hypersensitivity aetiology is thought likely and this is supported by the frequent association of fever, arthralgia, rash, peripheral eosinophilia and eosinophiluria. Oliguria, salt and potassium loss due to tubular dysfunction and modest proteinuria – are typical features. Some patients may be polyuric.

c) Full serum biochemical profile, including sodium, calcium, phosphate, and liver function test; full blood count – an eosinophilia is typical.

d) Renal ultrasound and biopsy. Renal biopsy typically shows a cellular infiltrate composed primarily of eosinophils, with superadded tubular necrosis. In some patients linear deposition of IgG and C3 along the tubular basement membrane has been shown.

e) Modification of the anti-TB treatment regime. Corticosteroids e.g. Prednisolone 60 mg/day, may lead to more rapid recovery of renal function. Correction of electrolyte imbalance is necessary and acute renal replacement therapy may be required. In most patients full recovery of renal function occurs.

Previous peritoneal TB is a contraindication to acute peritoneal dialysis, and haemodialysis would need to be performed on a unit accepting HBsAg-positive patients.

48 a) Non-sustained ventricular tachycardia.

b) None. The treatment of non-sustained ventricular tachycardia has not been shown to improve prognosis in heart failure.

c) Superior, (positive in lead 1 negative in II and III).

d) Atrial fibrillation. Ventricular tachycardia can result from digoxin toxicity, which is not uncommon in treated atrial fibrillation.

49 a) The patient is describing **two transient ischaemic attacks** involving the **carotid territory**. The visual symptoms are usually described as *amaurosis fugax*. The short duration, and nature of onset are typical – description of a blind or curtain coming across the field of vision is classical.

b) Has he experienced other attacks in the carotid territory, or in other vascular territories, e.g. vertebrobasilar, characterized by hemisensory disturbance or hemiparesis, diplopia, dizziness, nausea, ataxia, or dysarthria? Is there a relevant family history of stroke, or cardiac disease? Is there a history of smoking, hypertension, diabetes, angina, blackouts, claudication, or other systemic disease associated with arteritis? Were there any specific events that precipitated the attacks; any history of chest pain or palpitations, headache, sudden movement or anything to precipitate a fall in blood pressure (e.g. anti-hypertensive drugs)?

c) Lying and standing BP in both arms should be measured; bruits should be sought in all vascular territories; full cardiac examination, to exclude valvular pathology – about 30% of TIA patients have a potential cardiac source of embolism; splinter haemorrhages, other signs of endocarditis or evidence of a systemic vasculitis may sometimes be found; residual abnormal neurological signs are not generally found, but careful fundoscopy is required – platelet or cholesterol emboli may be present in the retinal arterioles.

d) The cause of the TIA should be sought – history and examination, as above, will often provide useful pointers. Relevant investigations are FBC, ESR, biochemical profile, blood glucose, fasting lipids, VDRL, urinalysis, CXR, ECG and CT scan. Echocardiography or 24-hour ECG monitoring may be appropriate. Digital subtraction angiography of the great vessels is appropriate in a young patient with suspected carotid disease, in whom surgery is being considered.

Medical treatment comprises; i) control of risk factors: BP, diabetes, hyperlipidaemia, obesity, smoking; ii) anti-platelet therapy with aspirin; iii) appropriate therapy for cardiac arrythmias, or valve disease if relevant.

e) Myocardial infarction.

50 a) The combination of thrombocytopenia, renal failure and cholestatic jaundice in a trout farmer is highly suggestive of **leptospirosis (Weil's disease)**. It is unusual for the other causes of jaundice such as viral hepatitis, infectious mononucleosis, malaria, Legionnaire's disease or brucellosis to present with this triad but these diagnoses should be actively excluded. Leptospirosis, a spirochaetal disease (caused by the *Leptospira interrogans* complex) is carried by rodents and usually passed to humans by contact with rat urine or blood, typically occurring in those exposed to rat excreta in the context of their occupation.

The clinical presentation varies from the classic picture of Weil's disease with multi-organ involvement, to a mild anicteric febrile illness. Clinical features include fever, lymphadenopathy, headache, photophobia, conjunctival injection, abdominal pain, splenomegaly and profound myalgia. Renal involvement occurs in approximately 50% of cases and varies from mild proteinuria to dialysis-dependent renal failure. Jaundice occurs in 10% of cases and is typically cholestatic. Pulmonary involvement is common, though the severity varies from a dry cough to marked pulmonary infiltration with respiratory failure.

b) The diagnosis of leptospirosis may be made in the first 10 days of the illness by culture of blood or cerebrospinal fluid. Urine cultures become positive from the 2nd week. Serological diagnosis is possible after the 10th day using a macroscopic slide agglutination test or rising antibody titres. A peripheral blood polymorphonuclear leucocytosis is usual.

The cerebrospinal fluid findings – a normal sugar, slightly elevated protein with a lymphocyte pleocytosis, though initially neutrophils may predominate.

c) Penicillin or tetracyclines should be given within the first 5 days of the illness. Supportive treatment with attention to fluid balance is essential. Dialysis may be necessary. Overall the prognosis is good; poor prognosis factors include severe jaundice, disseminated intravascular coagulation, renal failure and respiratory failure.

51 a) Rupture of the oesophagus. The occurrence of severe retrosternal chest pain in a hypertensive smoker is obviously suggestive of myocardial ischaemia. However, the radiation of cardiac pain to the back is unusual in an uncomplicated myocardial infarction and is more compatible with aortic dissection. Against the diagnosis of aortic dissection is the lack of pulse inequality, the absence of aortic incompetence and the presence of a left pleural effusion.

The history of pain starting during a meal, and radiating through to the back coupled with the presence of a left pleural effusion in a shocked patient, is highly suggestive of a ruptured oesophagus.

b) The diagnosis may be confirmed by gastrograffin examination of the oesophagus, which will demonstrate the presence of a tear.

52 a) Phenytoin toxicity presenting with cerebellar syndrome, mild megaloblastic anaemia and osteomalacia. The recent fit might be paradoxical, i.e. related to high phenytoin levels. Rifampicin is an enzyme inducer and unlikely to be responsible for high phenytoin levels unless the dosage of phenytoin had been increased to compensate.

b) Investigations should include measurement of plasma phenytoin level, serum folate and vitamin B_{12} and vitamin D levels.

The principal side-effects of phenytoin include:
1) Central nervous system – cerebellar signs, typically ataxia, tremor, nystagmus and dysarthria; sedation; mood swings; peripheral neuropathy; increased fits.
2) Haematological – folate deficiency leading to a megaloblastic anaemia; aplastic anaemia; lymphadenopathy.
3) Endocrine – increased metabolism of vitamin D which may lead to osteomalacia; reduced ADH levels, worsening of diabetes mellitus.
4) Skin – acne; coarsening of facial features; gum hypertrophy; Dupuytren's contractures.
5) Hepatitis.
6) Drug-induced LE.
7) Drug fever.
8) Fetal abnormalities – microcephaly, congenital heart disease, cleft palate and hare lip.

There is a large genetic variation in the rate of phenytoin metabolism, so that monitoring levels is essential. A number of drugs impair phenytoin metabolism, including isoniazid, chloramphenicol, and dicoumarol. Ethanol and carbamazepine increase phenytoin metabolism.

Note: Phenytoin is an enzyme inducer and will increase the metabolism of drugs such as the oral contraceptive pill.

53 A

a) Pulmonary vascular disease, e.g. multiple pulmonary emboli
Primary pulmonary hypertension
Right-to-left shunt

b) Echocardiogram; cardiac catheter

B

a) Pulmonary fibrosis secondary to rheumatoid arthritis.

b) CT scan, bronchoalveolar lavage, open lung biopsy.

54 a) Diplopia, aggressive/uninhibited behaviour, nystagmus, confusion, slurred speech, dehydration.

b) A history or signs of a head injury, e.g. skull fracture, subdural or extradural haemorrhage or other injury should be sought. Consider the possibility of ingestion of other drugs – e.g. barbiturates, heroin, antihistamines, methanol, ethylene glycol, cocaine, 'crack'. Look at the pupils, look for needle marks, talk to the police or to friends who may accompany the patient; consider hypoglycaemia or other metabolic upset.

c) Hypoglycaemia; rhabdomyolysis; fits; inhalation; peptic ulceration; pancreatitis; irreversible brain damage; liver failure; hallucinations/tremor; Wernicke's encephalopathy; and Korsakoff's psychosis.

d) Ensure that the patient's airway remains patent; keep him hydrated; be aware of the risks of hypoglycaemia; treat fits and withdrawal symptoms as required; Vitamin B replacement (primarily thiamine). Consider appropriate psychiatric assessment or specialist counselling if the problem is one of chronic alcohol abuse.

55 a) Benign intracranial hypertension. The syndrome of an
elevation in CSF pressure in the absence of ventricular dilation
or intracerebral mass.

Benign intracranial hypertension is predominantly a disease of
obese females. The aetiology is unknown though associations
with pregnancy, drugs (eg. tetracyclines, nalidixic acid), dural
sinus thrombosis, previous head injury and vitamin A deficiency
states have been noted. Neurological signs are usually confined
to swollen discs, though a partial VI nerve palsy is often found.
A space-occupying lesion must be excluded.

b) CT scan – the ventricles will not be displaced, and may be
normal or small. The diagnosis is confirmed by finding an
elevated cerebrospinal fluid pressure. Dural sinus thrombosis
should be excluded by angiography.

c) Visual loss due to optic atrophy. Permanent visual loss occurs
in up to 50% of cases and may be severe in 10%.

d) Weight loss and diuretics form the mainstay of treatment.
Initially therapeutic lumbar punctures may be performed and
high-dose corticosteroids have been used initially to reduce
intracranial pressure effectively. Surgery is not usually required,
though ventriculoperitoneal shunting of cerebrospinal fluid may
be needed if visual loss is progressive and the response to
steroids is slow.

Most cases undergo clinical remission either spontaneously or
in response to treatment, though CSF pressure may remain high.

56 a) In the presence of acute chest pain the anterior changes are
likely to represent left anterior descending (LAD) coronary artery
occlusion. There is an inferior infarct of indeterminate age which
probably results from right coronary artery occlusion.

b) The appearance of Q-waves early in an infarction is one
feature of thrombolysis.

c) The atrioventricular node is an inferior structure. Its
involvement in an anterior myocardial infarction is evidence of
an extensive area of damage and is a poor prognostic sign.

d) Persistent ST segment elevation at 1 year strongly suggests
the presence of a left ventricular aneurysm.

57 **a) Intracardiac right-to-left shunting.** The most marked effect of a shunt on saturation is in the chamber beyond that receiving the shunted blood; in this case that is the femoral artery, suggesting a ventricular septal defect.

b) There is a marked peak-to-peak systolic gradient across the pulmonary valve, indicating stenosis.

c) Overriding aorta. There is demonstrable ventricular septal defect, pulmonary stenosis and right ventricular hypertrophy; the most likely diagnosis is Fallot's tetralogy.

d) Dizzy spells may represent:

1) Increased right-to-left shunting with reduced peripheral vascular resistance (exercise) and therefore increasing systemic desaturation.
2) Recurrent paradoxical emboli are common due to polycythaemia and the right-to-left shunt.
3) Recurrent paroxysmal arrhythmias as a result of atrial distension.

58 **a) Multiple sclerosis** – retrobulbar neuritis.

b) Diminished acuity and colour vision in the affected eye, particularly centrally. Peripheral vision may be retained; the optic disc may be swollen. Examination of both eyes may reveal nystagmus and/or an internuclear ophthalmoplegia.

c) The episode of 'foot dragging' is explicable by the presence of a spinal cord plaque. Brainstem involvement often produces symptoms which may be confused with vestibular neuronitis. Such a relapsing/remitting course is typical of demyelinating disease.

d) Visual evoked responses; auditory evoked responses; CSF examination for evidence of local IgG synthesis; NMR scanning if available.

e) Acuity may return to normal over a few months, though there may be residual impairment of colour vision; recurrent attacks can occur. The temporal half of the optic disc (containing macular fibres) will be pale.

59 a) Hypocalcaemia due to hypoparathyroidism. The biochemical findings of hypocalcaemia with an elevated phosphate and a normal alkaline phosphatase (normal for an 8 year old) are typical.

b) The differential diagnosis includes primary hypoparathyroidism and pseudohypoparathyroidism (the typical phenotype of pseudohypoparathyroidism includes an oval face and short 4th and 5th metacarpal bones).

These may be differentiated by:

1) Measurement of serum PTH levels – absent in primary hypoparathyroidism, and present in pseudohypoparathyroidism, where the abnormality is a failure to respond to PTH.

2) The diagnosis of pseudohypoparathyroidism may be confirmed by the Ellsworth Howard test – a PTH infusion fails to increase urine phosphate and cyclic AMP, in contrast to primary hypoparathyroidism where both are elevated.

60 a) Hydralazine-induced lupus erythematosus. The clinical picture of rash, polyarthritis, pericarditis with pericardial effusion, pleural effusions, a positive ANA, raised ESR and leucopenia in a patient on hydralazine strongly suggests the diagnosis.

b) The hydralazine should be stopped. Remission following drug withdrawal is the rule, although this may take several months. Low-dose oral prednisolone will control her symptoms until the illness settles.

Drug-induced lupus erythematosus occurs more often in the elderly. The onset of the disease appears to be related to a cumulative effect. There is a strong genetic contribution for several drugs. Both slow acetylator status and the possession of the allele HLA DR4 increase the risk of hydralazine-induced lupus erythematosus. The clinical picture is similar to idiopathic lupus but renal and central nervous system disease are rare. The ANA may be positive with a high titre. However antibodies such as ds-DNA antibodies, found in idiopathic lupus, are unusual and present only in low titre. Antihistone antibodies, particularly against the H2 fraction are characteristic of drug-induced lupus erythematosus.

The commonest drugs implicated are procainamide, hydralazine, phenytoin, isoniazid and chlorpromazine. Rarely, β-blockers have been implicated.

61 a) There is a significant gradient between the left atrial pressure (pulmonary capillary wedge) and left ventricle at end-diastole, indicating mitral stenosis.

b) The A-wave is a measurement of pressure at peak atrial contraction. The most common cause of an exaggerated A-wave is a hypertrophied and thus poorly compliant ventricle. In this case the right ventricle is clearly hypertrophied in response to pulmonary arterial hypertension.

c) Three features of palpation:

1) A palpable impulse of mitral valve closure (first heart sound) – 'tapping apex.'

2) A left parasternal systolic heave (right ventricular hypertrophy).

3) A palpable impulse of pulmonary valve closure (second heart sound) at high left parasternal area, a consequence of pulmonary hypertension.

d) A-waves only occur with atrial contraction – therefore sinus rhythm.

62 a) The differential diagnosis is of a single pulmonary nodule associated with linear shadowing, and a granulomatous reaction. The most likely diagnosis in this case is chronic infection caused by **histoplasmosis**.
Histoplasma capsulatum may cause an acute pneumonia or chronic pulmonary lesions. In endemic areas (such as Southern USA) the majority of those exposed never develop overt signs of infection unless they become immunosuppressed. Bird and bat excreta may contain large numbers of the organisms, and a history of inhalation of dust from a cave containing bats (as in this case), or a bird-house, is often noted in acute histoplasmosis. The acute illness occurs 2–3 weeks after exposure. The radiological changes tend to be out of proportion to the relatively mild symptoms. Cultures are typically negative. A rising complement fixation titre confirms the diagnosis. The pneumonia often settles without treatment and when acute is unresponsive to conventional antibiotics. In severe cases intravenous amphotericin B is given. Acute re-infection may cause acute bilateral pulmonary infiltrates and breathlessness. Chronic pulmonary disease is unusual but is recognized especially in male smokers. Progressive disease requires amphotericin B. Coin lesions may cavitate, or more commonly calcify. Rarely, patients may present with mediastinitis and SVC obstruction, or disseminated disease.

b) The other possibilities include:

1) Malignancy: a primary carcinoma or a metastasis (colon, kidney, germ-cell, melanoma, prostate or bone are the most likely in a man of this age).
2) A hypersensitivity reaction and fibrosis related to dust inhalation. However, typically both lungs would be affected.
3) Wegener's granulomatosis restricted to the lungs may occur but is extremely rare.
4) A chronic infection with acid-fast bacilli is unlikely since the organism has not been detected and the tuberculin test is negative.
5) Sarcoidosis – this would be a very atypical presentation of sarcoidosis.

c) Further investigations should include i) complement fixation tests for fungi, particularly histoplasmosis and coccidioidomycosis; ii) culture of the biopsy material for fungi; the organisms may be difficult to detect even with specific stains in fibrosed material; iii) a thoracotomy and biopsy of the nodule to exclude malignancy and obtain material in which the yeasts should be easily seen using appropriate stains.

63 **a) Osteonecrosis (avascular necrosis) of the femoral head.** Head of the humerus, medial and lateral condyles of the distal femur, superior margin of the talus may also be affected.

b) Plain X-rays of both hips. The plain X-ray is often initially normal but may show an infarcted area with surrounding radiolucency, a sclerotic rim around the lesion, loose fragments of bone, or fractures.

An isotope bone scan is the test of choice and will initially show an area of reduced uptake which may be surrounded by increased tracer localization. As repair gets under way, or if there is extensive damage (with a fracture, for example) there may be generally increased uptake.

c) The patient received an excess of steroid. A more usual regimen would be hydrocortisone 20 mg *mane*, 10 mg *nocte*. High dose steroids are the most important cause of osteonecrosis, and in this patient may have contributed both directly and indirectly by causing weight gain.

Factors implicated in the pathogenesis of osteonecrosis include:

1) Trauma, e.g. fracture – called avascular necrosis
2) Excess corticosteroids
3) Sickle cell disease
4) Deep sea diving
5) Radiotherapy
6) Alcohol
7) Pregnancy
8) Rheumatic diseases, e.g. rheumatoid arthritis, systemic lupus erythematosus
9) Hereditary disorders, e.g. Fabry's disease, Gaucher's disease, hyperlipidaemia
10) Infection, e.g. infective endocarditis.

64A **a) Acute pancreatitis.** The low albumin, low corrected calcium, hypoxia and high blood glucose all point to the diagnosis, which may be confirmed by measurement of serum amylase levels; a level >1000 Somogyi units is said to be diagnostic.

b) Thiazide diuretics are a recognized cause of acute pancreatitis. Other drugs which may precipitate an acute attack include steroids, azathioprine and the contraceptive pill. In the UK the majority of cases of acute pancreatitis are idiopathic – the commonest-known precipitating cause is gallstones; other precipitating factors include alcohol, viral infections particularly mumps, trauma – which may be local e.g. following ERCP or following general surgery, carcinoma of the pancreas, hyperparathyroidism and hypertriglyceridaemia.

64B **a) Intracranial tumour**, localized probably to the frontal cortex.

b) A fit *de novo* in a patient of this age always raises the suspicion of a space-occupying lesion. A previous history of headaches is important. Intellectual impairment, mood change, particularly euphoric or impulsive behaviour, are all typical of frontal lobe lesions.

c) Most intracranial tumours are secondary; FBC, ESR, full biochemical screen, and chest X-ray should be performed, together with a CT brain scan.

65 **a) Thyroid crisis or thyroid storm**. There is a family history of autoimmune disease and a good history of progressive weight loss – an indication of hyperthyroidism. The acute deterioration followed an upper respiratory tract infection and the patient presented with the classic combination of i) fever;
ii) cardiovascular symptoms – arrhythmias and hypotension;
iii) neurological involvement – confusion, agitation; and
iv) gastrointestinal involvement with abdominal pain and vomiting.

b) The condition is a medical emergency.

Management steps: Intravenous β-blockers – propranolol 2 mg i.v. is effective in relieving fever and tachycardia. 20 mg of carbimazole by nasogastric tube, repeated 4-hourly, or an equivalent dosage of propylthiouracil.

In some centres sodium iodide is given 1 hour after the first dose of carbimazole to prevent further release of thyroid hormones.

General supportive treatment; intravenous fluids; the patient may need appropriate sedation and digoxin may be necessary to control the atrial fibrillation.

Blood should be sent for measurement of thyroid hormones and thyroid autoantibodies.

Answer to questions 66–67A

66 a) The antiphospholipid syndrome characterized by thrombosis, both arterial and venous, recurrent abortions and thrombocytopenia.

b) Antiphospholipid antibodies are immunoglobulins of the IgG and IgM class which are directed against negatively-charged phospholipid molecules. They were first described in systemic lupus erythematosus, but have since been described in a wide range of autoimmune diseases associated with a variety of autoantibodies, but can occur in isolation – the antiphospholipid syndrome.

A wide range of neurological diseases have been linked to the presence of antiphospholipid antibodies, including recurrent migraines, chorea and transient ischaemic attacks. Other associations include livedo reticularis, endocardial lesions and pulmonary hypertension.

c) The presence of antiphospholipid antibodies may be suggested by i) the presence of a lupus anticoagulant as indicated by a prolonged APTT which cannot be corrected by the addition of normal plasma; ii) the presence of a false positive VDRL.

Antiphospholipid antibodies are measured by a radioimmunoassay or ELISA – in specialist units.

Note: a negative VDRL or the absence of a lupus anticoagulant does not exclude the presence of antiphospholipid antibodies.

67A a) The combination of acute abdominal pain, vomiting, epilepsy and a predominant motor neuropathy suggest the diagnosis of **acute intermittent porphyria**. This diagnosis is further supported by the hyponatraemia, raised serum bilirubin and aspartate transaminase levels.

b) Measure i) urine-d-aminolaevulinic acid, and ii) urinary porphobilinogen. Both should be greatly raised during the acute attack; levels are also raised during remission. The addition of Ehrlich's aldehyde reagent to the urine should result in a pink colour due to the presence of porphobilinogen. A similar result is also obtained if the urine contains urobilinogen. The addition of n-butanol distinguishes porphobilinogen, which is insoluble in n-butanol, unlike urobilinogen which is soluble.

67B a) Galactosaemia (an autosomal recessive disorder): incidence 1:60 000 due to deficiency of the enzyme galactose-1-phosphate uridyl transferase. Deficiency of this enzyme results in high levels of galactose-1-phosphate which is thought to be responsible for organ damage.

b) Clinical features manifest soon after birth and include failure to thrive, vomiting, diarrhoea, hepatomegaly, jaundice, hypoglycaemia, cataracts, a Fanconi-type syndrome and psychomotor retardation. A well-recognized late complication, especially in girls, is hypergonadotropic hypogonadism.

c) The diagnosis should be confirmed by measuring erythrocyte enzyme levels of galactose-1-phosphate uridyl transferase activity. Blood and urine galactose levels are raised in this condition.

d) Galactose should be excluded from the diet, probably for life. In infancy a milk substitute such as Nutramigen may be used. Treatment should be monitored by measuring erythrocyte levels of galactose-1-phosphate.

68 a) The patient has a progressive neurological disorder involving the brainstem (by vertigo and tinnitus) and cerebellum (dysarthria, ataxia and nystagmus). She also has weight loss, ascites and a cystic lesion affecting the right ovary. CT scan shows cortical and cerebellar atrophy. The most likely diagnosis is a **paraneoplastic syndrome involving the cerebellum and brainstem**, associated with an **ovarian neoplasm**. Carcinoma of the bronchus is also a possibility but this patient was a non-smoker and the chest X-ray is normal apart from old tuberculous apical changes.

The CSF protein and cell count is raised, so the differential diagnosis should include chronic meningitis due to fungus, tuberculosis or carcinoma. However, such diseases typically cause cranial nerve palsies or focal problems due to infiltration or a mass effect. Lymphomas cause meningeal infiltration and are also associated with more frequent opportunistic infections of the central nervous system (Listeria, cryptoccocus, toxoplasma and fungi) which may have more diffuse effects.

Serum potassium is low, which can be explained by a combination of diuretics and poor diet.

b) The investigation of choice would be a laparotomy and removal of the ovaries for histology. Generally a total abdominal hysterectomy is performed, with sampling of the pelvic lymph nodes to stage the disease.

Paraneoplastic cerebellar–brainstem degeneration is most commonly associated with carcinoma of the ovary. Other tumours linked to the syndrome are breast, lung and Hodgkin's disease.

The central nervous system paraneoplastic syndromes tend to overlap with each other. The major groups include:
1) Cerebellar degeneration.
2) Limbic encephalitis (amnesia, hallucinations and epilepsy).
3) Lower brain stem encephalitis.
4) Spinal cord disease causing a pryamidal or extrapyramidal syndrome.
5) Degeneration of the dorsal root ganglia causing a sensory ataxia or anterior horn cell degeneration which may lead to a bulbar palsy.

How certain tumours cause selective neuronal death is not known. Antibodies to cells in the dorsal root ganglia and Purkinje cells have been identified, an observation consistent with an immunological mechanism. Treatment of paraneoplastic CNS-degenerations is rarely effective. Occasionally, removal of the primary neoplasm is followed by improvement.

69 A

a) Bilateral diaphragm weakness/paralysis.

b) Muscular dystrophy, surgical trauma to phrenic nerves, poliomyelitis, Pompe's glycogen storage disease (acid maltase deficiency).

B

a) Marked elevation in the KCO (NB this has been corrected for the Hb) suggesting alveolar haemorrhage, which can occur in the absence of frank haemoptysis.

b) Goodpasture's syndrome, Wegener's granulomatosis, microscopic polyarteritis, systemic lupus erythematosus.

C

a) Asthma.

70 a) The initial diagnosis of giant-cell arteritis was based on the clinical history, examination findings of tender carotid arteries and an elevated ESR. Giant-cell arteritis is a segmental panarteritis of unknown aetiology affecting large and medium-sized vessels. In most centres it is clinical practice to perform a temporal artery biopsy to confirm the diagnosis before commencing the patient on high-dose corticosteroids. Typically symptoms respond promptly to high doses of prednisolone and this is mirrored by a fall in the acute-phase response. In this case the patient failed to respond to treatment, which raises the possibility of a **paraneoplastic musculoskeletal syndrome**. These may take many forms and include myopathy, arthropathy, polymyalgia, giant-cell arteritis, scleroderma, polymyositis, and vasculitis. Clinically it is impossible to distinguish between true giant-cell arteritis and the paraneoplastic syndrome, but paraneoplastic syndromes tend to respond poorly to conventional doses of prednisolone.

b) A **renal cell carcinoma** needs to be excluded if the patient has haematuria and proteinuria. Renal cell carcinoma (hypernephroma) has a peak incidence in the 5th to 7th decades and occurs in males more commonly than females.

Renal cell carcinoma may have protean manifestations which include haematuria (55%), elevated ESR (55%), abdominal mass (45%), loin pain (41%), hypertension (35%), weight loss, fever, hypercalcaemia, erythrocytosis and musculoskeletal paraneoplastic syndromes.

71 a) Buerger's disease – the patient presented with a left popliteal
artery occlusion.
The differential diagnosis of an acute popliteal artery occlusion
lies between a thrombosis or an embolism. Against embolism is
the lack of a cardiac source – no bruits, no murmurs, a normal
ECG and echocardiogram (no atrial myxoma, thrombus,
aneurysm or abnormal valves), and no history of arrhythmias. A
small percentage of emboli may arise from a source in a
peripheral artery, but the proximal vessels in the arteriogram
were normal.
Thrombosis may be the result of:
1) Abnormal clotting stages: e.g. antithrombin III deficiency,
   myeloproliferative disorders, etc.
2) Compression narrowing the lumen.
3) Diseases which cause local damage to the wall of the vessel,
   e.g. Buerger's disease, cryoglobulinaemia (associated with
   purpura and cutaneous gangrene), atherosclerosis and
   vasculitis (primary, associated with a connective tissue disease
   or a malignancy).
The lack of systemic symptoms, the laboratory results (mild
acute phase response only) the distribution of the vessels
involved and the appearance of the arteriogram make Buerger's
disease or thrombo-angitis obliterans the most likely diagnosis.
This condition typically affects males below 30 years of age; it is
very rare in women and thought not to occur in non-smokers.
Buerger's disease is characterized by occlusion of small and
medium-sized vessels, thrombophlebitis and Raynaud's
phenomenon. Histologically there is a localized panarteritis which
leads to thrombosis. Arteriograms often show otherwise normal
vessels with 'corrugations' in the vessel immediately proximal to
the obstruction, distinguishing the condition from pre-senile
atherosclerotic arterial obstruction. Typically there is no, or only
a mild, acute phase response.
b) Treatment of an acute thrombotic episode is thrombolysis,
followed by arterial grafts if dissolution of the clot fails or
claudication remains a significant symptom. To prevent
recurrence, total abstinence from smoking is essential.
c) Further investigations should include: histology of the clot if
thrombolysis fails, which typically contains granulomas and
neutrophils in Burger's disease, or an arterial wall biopsy to
demonstrate neutrophil infiltration of all layers of the vessel wall.

72 This patient is in **cardiogenic shock**.

a) The cyanosis in the presence of fully saturated arterial blood arises from poor peripheral perfusion.

b) Blood flow (cardiac output) is poor and therefore there is greater than normal oxygen extraction at the tissues from each passage of blood through the capillary beds. Inferior vena cava blood is always of lower saturation because hepatic venous blood is extremely desaturated.

c) The high V-wave in the PCWP suggests some mitral regurgitation. This is probably secondary to left ventricular dilation and dysfunction, in which case there is no benefit from surgery. If, however, there is primary mitral valve disease (e.g. damage due to endocarditis) there may be considerable haemodynamic improvement from mitral valve replacement.

d) The arterial blood is fully saturated. The high wedge pressure in the absence of pulmonary arterial hypertension suggests that the pulmonary venous hypertension is relatively acute, and should cause severe pulmonary oedema at this level. The maintenance of full saturation therefore suggests that the patient is receiving inspired oxygen therapy.

73 a) Primary biliary cirrhosis. The patient presents with a cholestatic hepatitis, hepatosplenomegaly, and an upper gastrointestinal haemorrhage. In addition she has an elevated serum IgM and her calcium is at the lower limit of normal (corrected Ca 2.0 mmol/l for an albumin) with a low serum phosphate suggesting early osteomalacia. Patients with primary biliary cirrhosis tend to have few stigmata of chronic liver disease compared with alcoholic liver disease or chronic active hepatitis.

b) Further investigations should include upper gastrointestinal endoscopy to distinguish between a peptic ulcer and bleeding varices (enlarged spleen suggests portal hypertension), anti-mitochondrial antibodies and a liver biopsy to confirm the diagnosis of primary biliary cirrhosis, and vitamin D level to evaluate the low calcium.

Primary biliary cirrhosis chiefly affects females between 30 and 60 years of age, and is second only to alcohol as a cause of chronic liver disease in such patients. Primary biliary cirrhosis may present with deranged liver function tests, pruritus, jaundice, abdominal pain, anorexia, weight loss, diarrhoea, osteopenia (and bone pain), and evidence of liver failure or upper gastrointestinal bleeding (increased incidence of peptic ulceration). Xanthelasma are common and chronic cases may be clubbed. The natural history is variable: asymptomatic patients may never develop significant disease. Symptomatic patients, e.g. those who present with pruritus, generally progress to cirrhosis with portal hypertension over 7–10 years. Why some patients have a non-progressive form of primary biliary cirrhosis is unknown.

The alkaline phosphatase and γ-GT are raised in >99% of patients; the alanine transaminase and aspartate aminotransferase are usually normal. Bilirubin rises late and suggests a poor prognosis. An elevated IgM is found in 80%, IgG in 40% and IgA only rarely.

Antimitochondrial antibodies are positive in >90% of cases; the titre does not have prognostic significance; only four antimitochondrial antibodies M2, M4, M8 (associated with a worse prognosis) and anti-M9 are associated with primary biliary cirrhosis. Anti-smooth muscle antibody or a weakly positive antinuclear factor are also common. A strongly positive anti-smooth muscle antibody or ANA is associated with disease with features of both chronic active Lupoid hepatitis and primary biliary cirrhosis.

Histologically the disease is patchy. The earliest lesion is a T-cell mediated focal damage to the interlobular bile ducts with associated granuloma formation, followed by bile duct obliteration/proliferation, fibrosis and finally cirrhosis.

Pruritus may be treated with cholestyramine, antihistamines, or if these fail, rifampicin or UV-radiation; rarely, haemoperfusion is necessary. Liver transplantion is now firmly established as treatment for end-stage primary biliary cirrhosis. D-penicillamine may produce an improvement in the short term but it is not sustained. Prednisolone improves the biochemical picture but increases osteopenia, hence should only be used with caution. Osteomalacia may be prevented with calcium and vitamin D supplements. Occasionally the other fat-soluble vitamins are reduced and cause symptoms – vitamin K (bruising), vitamin E (neuropathy), and vitamin A (night blindness). High cholesterol levels will require dietary modification.

74 a) A megaloblastic anaemia caused by failure of B_{12} absorption is the most likely diagnosis. The patient has previously undergone emergency surgery for abdominal pain and peritonism, raising the possibility of small bowel resection and/or the blind loop syndrome.

The first part of the Schilling test demonstrates malabsorption of vitamin B_{12}. The purpose of the second part of the test is to assess whether this defect is reversed by simultaneous administration of intrinsic factor. Correction of the malabsorption by intrinsic factor is almost diagnostic of pernicious anaemia. Failure of intestinal absorption is indicated if intrinsic factor fails to reverse the defect.

In blind loop syndromes, B_{12} deficiency is caused by bacterial utilization; the bacteria synthesize folate and the low B_{12} is often matched by a paradoxically high serum folate level.

b) Further investigations should include i) a small-bowel enema to exclude fistulae, strictures and blind loops, ii) quantitative bacterial analysis on jejunal aspirates and iii) a bile acid breath test.

Bile acid breath test – a radiolabelled ^{14}C conjugated bile acid is given orally and the amount of radioactive carbon dioxide excreted in the breath is measured along with faecal radioactivity. In normal individuals the conjugated bile acid is reabsorbed intact in the terminal ileum and little deconjugation occurs. In bacterial overgrowth affecting the small intestine, the bile acid is rapidly deconjugated and radioactive CO_2 excreted in the breath.

In disease of the terminal ileum, the bile acid is not absorbed and enters the colon where colonic bacterial deconjugate it, leading to radioactive CO_2 production. In ileal disease, unlike bacterial overgrowth, faecal excretion of radioactivity is high.

Causes of B_{12} deficiency include:

1) Nutritional
   Vegans
2) Gastric causes
   Addisonian pernicious anaemia, congenital deficiency of intrinsic factor, gastrectomy (partial or total) and atrophic gastritis.
3) Intestinal causes
   Blind loop syndrome, ileal resection, Crohn's disease, tropical sprue, fish tapeworm, transcobalamin 11 deficiency.
4) Drugs
   Para-aminosalicylic acid, colchicine, alcohol, biguanides.

Answer to questions 75-76

75 a) The tiredness and cold peripheries are likely to be related to the β-**blocker,** which needs to be either reduced or slowly withdrawn. The fluid retention is caused by the **oestrogen effect of fosfestrol,** which is metabolized to stilboestrol. The high T4 is likely to reflect high thyroxine binding globulin levels induced by stilboestrol. Thyrotoxicosis with symptoms suppressed by atenolol is not likely since the TSH is still within the normal range.

b) Measurement of thyroid binding globulin and the free T4 would be the most appropriate investigations.

76 a) i) **Sub-arachnoid haemorrhage.**
 ii) Meningitis.
Subarachnoid haemorrhage (SAH) is most likely. The patient gives a history of a headache of acute onset – typical of subarachnoid haemorrhage – and is apyrexial.

b) Lumbar puncture (provided no evidence of raised intracranial pressure).
Organisms and/or an elevated WBC and low glucose count point to a diagnosis of meningitis; frankly bloody fluid or xanthochromia (if the tap is performed after 24–48 hours) indicate subarachnoid haemorrhage.
Note: 48 hours after a subarachnoid haemorrhage there may be a reactive cerebrospinal fluid leucocytosis and low sugar.

c) CT scan when possible, full blood count, plasma glucose, clotting profile, blood cultures, CSF culture, routine urea and electrolytes.

d) Ruptured intracranial aneurysm. The commonest sites are the anterior communicating artery 30%, middle carotid artery 25% and posterior communicating 25%; 15% have multiple aneurysms; 5% bleed from arteriovenous malformations.

e) Acutely – the exclusion of meningitis, rest, analgesia ± antiemetic agents, careful monitoring of neurological state, and control of BP are important.
   Diagnosis can be made by CT scanning if available, but lumbar puncture is always indicated if there is any suspicion of meningitis. Referral to a neurosurgical centre for angiography is indicated – rebleeds commonly occur at around 1 week, and may be fatal. If technically possible, surgical clipping of an aneurysm is performed. If no lesion is identified at angiography, management is conservative.

77 a) The differential diagnosis of a unilateral mass on the chest X-ray and a slowly progressive paraparesis would include primary chest carcinoma with spinal secondaries, lymphoma with spinal deposits, infection e.g. tuberculosis, and sarcoidosis. The elevated serum calcium and low corrected transfer factor favour a diagnosis of **sarcoidosis**, though malignancy cannot be excluded. The hypochromic microcytic anaemia can be explained by the patient's menorrhagia.

b) As a matter of urgency a thoracic myelogram should be performed to exclude cord compression. Other relevant investigations are:

Neurological tests: CT head scan, NMR scans of head, cervical and thoracic spines, CSF examination.

Tests to obtain a tissue diagnosis: CT chest scan, fibreoptic bronchoscopy combined with biopsy or lavage, anterior mediastinoscopy and node biopsy.

Miscellaneous: Serum angiotensin-converting enzyme and Kveim test, serum iron and total iron binding capacity.

In this patient the diagnosis of sarcoidosis was confirmed by finding non-caseating granulomas on blind mucosal biopsy and on lymph node biopsy at mediastinoscopy. The thoracic myelogram and head CT scan were normal but NMR scans showed extensive confluent areas of high signal from the periventricular areas of the brain and upper cervical cord, suggestive of neurosarcoidosis.

Neurosarcoidosis complicates 5% of cases of sarcoidosis and may be the presenting manifestation of sarcoidosis in these patients. Neurosarcoidosis may have protean manifestations and can present with new clinical signs over a prolonged period of time and hence may mimic multiple sclerosis.

Neurosarcoidosis for simplicity may be divided into
i) neuropathies involving cranial and/or peripheral nerves (VII most commonly involved), and ii) CNS sarcoidosis involving the meninges, brain and spinal cord.

Symptoms and signs include epilepsy, raised intracranial pressure, hypothalamic syndromes, low grade meningitis, pyramidal signs, brainstem syndromes. Sarcoid granulomatous infiltrates in the cervical cord tend to affect primarily the pyramidal tracts.

Prognostically, cases of neurosarcoidosis can be divided into 2 groups: i) those with a monophasic illness who tend to respond well to high-dose prednisolone and have a good outcome, and ii) those with a chronic or relapsing course, in general responding poorly to prednisolone.

Note: i) Oligoclonal bands may be found in the CSF of cases of neurosarcoidosis; ii) 2% of patients with sarcoidosis have unilateral hilar lymphadenopathy.

78A a) A glucagonoma. Glucagonomas are alpha-cell pancreatic tumours which secrete glucagon and other related pancreatic peptides. They are present in adult life and are more common in females than males. Patients typically present with a necrolytic migratory rash and diabetes mellitus; other features include weight loss, diarrhoea and venous thrombosis.

b) The diagnosis is confirmed by finding elevated fasting plasma glucagon levels.

c) Surgical excision is the treatment of choice, and if removal is complete, is associated with complete resolution of symptoms. Many of these tumours are, however, widely disseminated at the time of diagnosis. Streptozotocin may be used to reduce metastasis size and symptoms; arterial embolization may be used to treat hepatic secondaries. The diabetes is usually insulin-dependent, anticoagulation will reduce the risk of thrombosis and oral zinc supplements may help the rash.

78B a) Primary hyperaldosteronism – Conn's syndrome – due to an adrenal adenoma or adrenal hyperplasia. The combination of hypertension with the biochemical picture of hypernatraemia, hypokalaemia and a high serum bicarbonate concentration is typical. Hypertension and hypokalaemic alkalosis are also seen with ectopic ACTH production but the glucose level is usually elevated.

b) The diagnosis is confirmed by high serum aldosterone levels in the presence of low renin levels. The hypertension is typically resistant to ACE inhibitors. Arteriography and venous sampling, CT scanning, and cholesterol scanning are used to localize the source of aldosterone prior to surgery.

79 a) The disorder is **familial hypophosphataemic rickets**, inherited in an **X-linked dominant manner**. Tubular resorption of phosphate is defective leading to low plasma phosphate levels. Phosphate deficiency is the primary cause of the osteomalacia, which is characterized in these patients by a raised ALP but usually a normal or minimally-reduced plasma calcium concentration. Since the calcium is relatively normal there is rarely evidence of hyperparathyroidism. The diagnosis may be confirmed by showing an inappropriate phosphaturia.

Treatment is large doses of phosphate and if necessary a small dose of vitamin D.

b) A has a 50% chance of being affected.

B will be unaffected (mother has two normal X chromosomes).

80 The combination of acute onset neurological abnormalities in association with microangiopathic haemolytic anaemia disseminated intravascular coagulation, thrombocytopenia, and renal failure is highly suggestive of **thrombotic thrombocytopenic purpura**.

Thrombotic thrombocytopenic purpura is a disorder of unknown aetiology which primarily affects young females. Typically there is sudden onset of fever, neurological signs, evidence of bleeding and renal failure of varying severity. It is closely related to the haemolytic uraemic syndrome of childhood though neurological involvement is much commoner. Pathophysiologically the initial event is believed to be blood vessel endothelial cell damage which subsequently triggers the clotting cascade leading to platelet consumption and fibrin deposition, the latter damaging red blood cells producing the classical fragmented or helmet cells. Histologically there is widespread evidence of microvascular hyaline thrombi.

Treatment is difficult, in view of the grave prognosis corticosteroids, immunosuppressive agents, immunoglobulin infusions and plasma exchange have been used with varying success. Anticoagulation is sometimes judiciously used in an effort to halt the consumptive coagulopathy its possible beneficial effects being balanced against the risk of haemorrhage.

Microangiopathic haemolytic anaemia describes the mechanical destruction of red blood cells which arises secondary to changes in small blood vessels which include: microthrombi, fibrinoid necrosis and malignant cell infiltration. The blood film typically shows microspherocytes and fragmented red cells. Many patients with a microangiopathic haemolytic anaemia also have evidence of disseminated intravascular coagulation but the two disorders may occur separately and do not necessarily overlap. A reduced platelet count suggests an associated disseminated intravascular coagulation.

Causes of microangiopathic haemolytic anaemia include:

Septicaemia – e.g. meningococcal septicaemia
Haemolytic uraemic syndrome
Thrombotic thrombocytopenic purpura
Malignant hypertension
Pre-eclampsia
Renal cortical necrosis
Acute glomerulonephritis
Disseminated mucinous carcinomatosus.
Polyarteritis nodosa
Wegener's granulomatosis
SLE

81 a) No. Pulmonary oedema will usually occur when pulmonary venous pressure exceeds 25 mmHg. Orthopnoea will occur at lower pressures, therefore this patient will experience breathlessness on lying flat.

b) i) Ventriculoseptal defect.
ii) Acute mitral regurgitation.

c) Measurement of oxygen saturation of blood from the right atrial and pulmonary arterial ports of the Swan–Ganz catheter. If there is a ventriculoseptal defect the pulmonary artery blood will be significantly more saturated than right atrial blood.

d) Inspiration causes a reduction in intrathoracic pressure. The pulmonary veins are exclusively intrathoracic and inspiration will reduce pulmonary venous pressure and aid pulmonary venous return. Left ventricular stroke volume will be reduced and hence the flow of blood either across the mitral valve or ventriculoseptal defect in systole will be reduced, leading to a reduction in murmur intensity.

82 a) This man has evidence of **pituitary failure**, possibly as a result of his head injury. He has a low T4 but no compensatory rise in TSH; he has lost axillary and pubic hair, suggesting hypogonadism; he is pale, has a low sodium and postural hypotension features of ACTH deficiency.
Note: ACTH deficiency does not cause significant hyponatraemia, so typical of primary adrenal failure, since aldosterone is still secreted normally. There is however a dilutional hyponatraemia and postural hypotension due to cortisol deficiency.

b) Investigations should include i) measurement of pituitary hormones (TSH, ACTH, FSH, LH, GH, PRL), ii) measurement of other target hormones (T4, testosterone and cortisol), iii) a CT head scan to image the pituitary fossa, and iv) dynamic pituitary function tests to distinguish between pituitary and hypothalamic dysfunction (insulin-induced hypoglycaemia, and administration of TRH and GnRH).

c) Replacement therapy consists of hydrocortisone, oral thyroxine and depot testosterone. Thyroid replacement should be introduced under careful supervision in view of the history of ischaemic heart disease. Thyroxine should be started in low dosage and there is an argument for initially starting liothyronine in view of its shorter half life should angina be precipitated.
An explanation of the patient's therapy should emphasize that the treatment is for life and that the cortisol dose should be increased during illness.

83 a) The commonest cause of a Coombs' negative haemolytic anaemia is **hereditary spherocytosis** (an autosomal dominant disorder).

Haemolysis is indicated by reticulocytosis, absent haptoglobins and a raised bilirubin. The history suggestive of recurrent haemolysis, the family history of anaemia and splenomegaly are all compatible with this diagnosis.

The blood film shows microspherocytes and the diagnosis may be confirmed by demonstrating the increased red cell osmotic fragility caused by the hereditary red cell membrane abnormality.

A full family study should then be performed on the direct relatives of patients with this disorder. Splenectomy is usually performed in all cases, though it is usually delayed until 5 years of age because of the increased risk of infection (especially pneumococcal). Prophylactic daily penicillin and pneumococcal vaccination are recommended post-splenectomy.

84 a) A right deep venous thrombosis consequent upon **paroxysmal nocturnal haemoglobinuria**.

b) i) A right venogram.
   ii) Ham's test (acid lysis test), which measures the sensitivity of red blood cells to complement lysis.

The occurrence of a thrombotic episode in a patient with pancytopenia is highly suggestive of paroxysmal nocturnal haemoglobinuria (PNH). In this patient PNH is also suggested by the history of dark urine passed early in the morning, and intermittent abdominal pain. Paroxysmal nocturnal haemoglobinuria is an acquired clonal disorder characterized by a membrane abnormality which results in increased sensitivity to complement. It sometimes develops during the recovery phase of an acute aplastic anaemia. Clinically there is intermittent, classically nocturnal, haemolysis leading to dark urine. The haemolysis may be profound and life threatening. The mechanism of the thrombotic tendency is not clear but may reflect the susceptibility of platelets to complement activation. Other important sites for thrombosis include hepatic vein obstruction, producing the Budd-Chiari syndrome, and cerebral thrombosis. The episodes of abdominal pain are thought to result from episodes of thrombosis affecting small portal blood vessels.

The severity of the symptoms varies; some patients require regular blood transfusions. Corticosteroids and androgens have been used in an effort to control the degree of haemolysis, and iron supplements are necessary as a result of the considerable haemosiderinuria. Anticoagulation is necessary for thrombotic episodes. In some patients the condition is self-limiting as the abnormal clone disappears. Allogeneic bone marrow transplantation has been successfully performed in patients with severe disease.

85 An incomplete urine collection.
In this patient, at first glance the Schilling test is suggestive of terminal ileal Crohn's disease as the cause of the malabsorption – the addition of intrinsic factor does not increase B_{12} absorption. However, the urinary creatinine is too low for a male of average weight with grossly normal renal function. The calculated glomerular filtration rate from the above figures is 60.

$$GFR = \frac{[Creatinine]\ urine \times 24\ hour\ urine\ vol}{[Creatinine]\ plasma \times 1440} = 60\ mls/min$$

A glomerular filtration rate of 60 mls/min is compatible with a normal serum urea and creatinine but strongly suggests that the patient has only collected approximately 50% of his 24 hour urine output.

The $^{14}CO_2$ breath test provides confirmatory evidence that the low B_{12} is due to bacterial overgrowth and not terminal ileal disease.

86A a) The severe microcytosis in the absence of anaemia in a patient of appropriate ethnic origin is highly suggestive of either alpha or beta thalassaemia cell trait. The elevated Hb A2 >3.5% and Hb F are diagnostic of **beta thalassaemia trait**. Haemoglobin electrophoresis is normal in cases of alpha thalassaemia and alpha/beta chain synthesis ratio studies are needed for diagnosis.

b) The patient should be reassured that he will remain entirely asymptomatic. However it is vitally important that he and his partner are counselled about the implications of parenthood; if they are planning to have children his partner should be investigated for thalassaemia trait. If both are beta thalassaemia trait positive there is a 25% chance that one of their offspring will have beta thalassaemia major; this can be detected antenatally.

86B a) Chronic renal failure. Chronic renal failure explains the mild hyperkalaemia and acidosis, the hypocalcaemia and the normochromic normocytic anaemia. Most patients with chronic renal failure will have a low T4 and T3 but a normal TSH and TRH response. The T4 tends to normalize once effective renal replacement therapy is introduced.

Causes of galactorrhoea include:

1) Pregnancy
2) Antidopaminergic drugs
   phenothiazines
   butyrophenones
   metoclopramide
   methyldopa
3) Oestrogens
4) Hypothalamic/pituitary lesions
5) Hypothyroidism
6) Chronic renal failure
7) Ectopic prolactin secretion, e.g. bronchogenic carcinoma, hypernephroma.

87 a) Primary adrenal failure – the biochemical picture of hyponatraemia, hyperkalaemia, a moderately increased urea, and hypoglycaemia is typical. Moderate corrected hypercalcaemia is also a recognized feature of adrenal failure.

The low T4 raises the possibility of secondary adrenal failure but the increased TSH indicates normal pituitary function. A low T4 and high TSH are frequently seen in Addison's disease in the absence of functional hypothyroidism and revert to normal following steroid replacement.

Addison's disease in the Western world is most commonly autoimmune in nature and is associated with autoimmune hypothyroidism in approximately 10% of cases. In this case, the absence of thyroid antibodies and the patient's race puts tuberculosis higher on the list of causes of adrenal failure.

The diagnosis may be confirmed by:-

1) The short synacthen test – 250 mg of tetracosactrin is administered followed by measurement of cortisol levels at 0, 30 and 60 minutes. Failure of cortisol to increase by 250 nmol/l at 30 minutes to a level greater than 550 nmol/l confirms the diagnosis.
2) Measurement of ACTH levels – elevated in primary adrenal failure.
3) Abdominal X-ray – evidence of adrenal calcification with tuberculous adrenal destruction.
4) Measurement of adrenal autoantibodies.

b) Glucocorticoid replacement, typically hydrocortisone 20 mg *mane* and 10 mg *nocte*. Mineralocorticoid replacement with fludrocortisone 0.1 mg od. may be necessary.

88 **a) Coronary artery atherosclerosis.** ST segment depression extending from lead V3 to V6 of greater than 2 mm suggests ischaemia in the region supplied by the left anterior descending artery.

    b) The QRS complexes in the V leads demonstrate the voltage criteria for left ventricular hypertrophy. In the absence of systemic hypertension, aortic stenosis must be considered. This may cause exercise-induced ischaemia without coronary artery disease.

    c) i) Echocardiography to exclude aortic stenosis.

       ii) Coronary arteriography.

89A **a)** The clinical picture is one of a right femoral nerve lesion in a patient with a prolonged prothrombin time. The most likely diagnosis is a **psoas bleed** causing **femoral nerve compression** due to **over-anticoagulation** with **warfarin**. The recent change in drug treatment is the most likely culprit – amiodarone typically potentiates the effect of warfarin.

    The diagnosis of a psoas bleed may be confirmed by ultrasound or CT scan. The coagulopathy should urgently be reversed by infusion of fresh frozen plasma. Vitamin K is a competitive antagonist of warfarin and will correct the prolonged prothrombin time. However vitamin K is contraindicated in a patient with a prosthetic valve since it may be difficult to re-anticoagulate for several days.

89B **a)** The presence of a macrocytic anaemia, neutropenia and thrombocytopenia suggests a diagnosis of **myelodysplasia**. This diagnosis is supported by the presence of Pelger cells and circulating blasts. It is now recognized that there is a 7–10-fold increase in the incidence of acute myeloid leukaemia after intensive chemotherapy for Hodgkin's disease. These leukaemias are usually preceded by myelodysplasia. The risk of developing leukaemia is greatest 5 years after treatment but remains high for up to 8 years after the last course of chemotherapy. An increased risk of acute myeloid leukaemia also occurs in other diseases such as myeloma, polycythaemia rubra vera and carcinoma of the ovary and breast where alkylating agents are used. Such secondary leukaemias are associated with particular karyotypes such as 5q–. The long arm of chromosome 5 encodes a series of haemopoietic growth factors and differentiation antigens, and its deletion raises fascinating questions concerning the mechanism of secondary leukaemia.

    Immunosuppression with non-alkylating agents, as in recipients of renal or cardiac transplantation, is associated with an increased risk of non-Hodgkin's lymphoma.

90 **a)** There is an obvious delta wave which is positive in lead V1. This is **Wolff–Parkinson–White syndrome type A**.
b) i) A re-entrant supraventricular tachycardia.
ii) Atrial fibrillation.
The danger of atrial fibrillation is that the accessory path may be capable of conducting very fast atrial rates, leading to a fast ventricular response which may degenerate into ventricular arrhythmias.
c) Posterior myocardial infarction
Right bundle branch block
Right ventricular hypertrophy
Dextrocardia
Duchenne's muscular dystrophy.

91A **a) Autoimmune haemolytic anaemia complicating chronic lymphatic leukaemia.** The presence of lymphocytosis with lymphadenopathy and splenomegaly in this age group is very suggestive of chronic lymphatic leukaemia. Anaemia in chronic lymphatic leukaemia may be caused by marrow infiltration, hypersplenism or an autoimmune haemolytic anaemia. In this patient the polychromasia, spherocytosis, reticulocytosis and absent haptoglobins point to a diagnosis of haemolysis.
b) Direct Coomb's test. About 20% of patients with chronic lymphatic leukaemia will develop a positive Coombs' test at some time during their illness but only one third will develop significant haemolysis.
The haemolysis responds well to steroids and chlorambucil.

Answer to question 91B

91B a) The coagulation tests show a prolonged activated partial thromboplastin time (APTT) but normal prothrombin time (PT), indicating an abnormality of the intrinsic pathway of coagulation. The commonest cause of such an abnormality is factor VIII: C deficiency – **haemophilia A**, an X-linked recessive condition.

Factor IX deficiency – Haemophilia B/Christmas disease (X-linked R) will also produce the same abnormal clotting profile but its incidence is one fifth that of haemophilia A. Severe factor VIII deficiency (<1% normal levels) causes impaired generation of thrombin and results in bleeding into major weight-bearing joints and prolonged bleeding after surgery or dental extraction. Intracranial bleeding is the commonest cause of death in severe untreated haemophilia; other common sites of bleeding include the renal tract, muscles, subperiosteal region and the iliopsoas sheath. The severity of symptoms depends on the extent of factor VIII: C deficiency.

Primary haemostasis, which is caused by a combination of vasoconstriction and platelet aggregation, is normal in haemophilia A and B and there is no abnormality in the initial haemostatic response. The diagnosis may be confirmed by demonstrating a deficiency of factor VIII:C and normal levels of factor IX and X.

Note: In von Willebrand's disease (autosomal D inheritance) abnormal platelet function is associated with low factor VIII:C and VIIIR: AG activity. The following tests are abnormal prolonged APTT (may be normal), prolonged bleeding time and impaired ristocetin-induced platelet aggregation.

92 **a) Primary hyperparathyroidism** – approximately 83% of cases are due to a single adenoma, diffuse gland hyperplasia accounts for approximately 10% and multiple adenoma for 4% of cases.

Investigations show hypercalcaemia, a low phosphate, a raised alkaline phosphatase, and a hyperchloraemic metabolic acidosis. The elevated blood urea may be explained by dehydration subsequent to the polyuria induced by the hypercalcaemia. There is a well-recognized association between primary hyperparathyroidism and peptic ulceration which explains the epigastric pain (note: a gastrointestinal bleed could also account for the elevated urea).

b) Most patients with primary hyperparathyroidism are diagnosed on routine screening and are asymptomatic.

Clinical features include abdominal pain, renal colic, constipation, vomiting, polydypsia, polyuria, weakness, psychiatric changes, band keratopathy, peptic ulceration and pancreatitis. Fifty percent of patients with primary hyperparathyroidism will develop renal stones.

Note the association of i) primary hyperparathyroidism, pituitary tumours, pancreatic tumours and adrenal cortical tumours multiple-endocrine neoplasia type I (MEN Type I), and ii) primary hyperparathyroidism, medullary carcinoma of the thyroid, phaeochromocytomas, carcinoid tumours and mucosal neuromas (MEN Type II).

c) The diagnosis is confirmed by finding an inappropriately high parathyroid hormone level for the serum calcium. Other features of primary hyperparathyroidism include:

1) a hyperchloraemic metabolic acidosis (unlike other cases of hypercalcaemia.
2) elevated 24-hour urinary calcium excretion.
3) elevated urinary cAMP.
4) elevated urinary hydroxyproline excretion.
5) radiology: subperiosteal bone resorption, bone cysts, brown tumours and deformities.
6) the hydrocortisone suppression test fails to suppress calcium levels in primary hyperparathyroidism but does so in other cases of hypercalcaemia.

d) Causes of hypercalcaemia include:

1) Malignancy	8) Hyperthyroidism
2) Multiple myeloma	9) Adrenal failure
3) Primary hyperparathyroidism	10) Immobility with Paget's
4) Tertiary hyperparathyroidism	disease
5) Sarcoidosis	11) Phaeochromocytoma
6) Vitamin D toxicity	12) Thiazide diuretics.
7) Milk–alkali syndrome	

93 a) Polymyositis is the most likely diagnosis despite the normal muscle biopsy. Criteria for the diagnosis of polymyositis include:

1) symmetrical proximal muscle weakness
2) typical EMG changes
3) typical muscle biopsy
4) elevated serum muscle enzymes
5) skin changes of dermatomyositis.

Difficulty in climbing stairs is an early symptom of proximal muscle weakness and this is often accompanied by pain and stiffness.

Muscle enzymes (aspartate aminotransferase and creatinine phosphokinase) are raised and the EMG changes are typical. Approximately 20% of muscle biopsies are negative as the disease is often patchy in its distribution.

The erythrocyte sedimentation rate and serum immunoglobulins are often elevated, as in this case.

The autoantibodies anti-Jo1, anti-P17 and anti-P112 are found in a subset of polymyositis patients who develop pulmonary fibrosis.

Clinical investigations to detect occult malignancy should be considered in patients over the age of 50.

94 a) Investigation was performed during the investigation of suspected **acromegaly**.

b) Two diagnoses may be made:

i) the patient is acromegalic: baseline growth hormone levels are elevated and fail to suppress with an oral glucose tolerance test.
ii) the patient is also diabetic.

Whole blood glucose values are 10–15% less than plasma. Capillary values are approximately 8% greater than venous values.

Diagnostic values for 750 g oral glucose tolerance test (in 250 ml water):

Venous Whole Blood	Fasting mmol/l	Two hours post oral GTT mmol/l
Normal	<6.7	<6.7
Diabetes mellitus	≥6.7	≥10
Impaired glucose tolerance	<6.7	>6.7 ≤10

Venous plasma	Fasting mmol/l	Two hours post oral GTT mmol/l
Normal	<7.8	<7.8
Diabetes mellitus	≥7.8	≥11.1
Impaired glucose tolerance	<7.8	>7.8 ≤11.1

95A a) Aluminium toxicity.

b) First stop aluminium hydroxide and use non-aluminium containing phosphate binder as necessary. Definitive treatment involves intravenous desferrioxamine. Patients with end-stage renal failure are at risk of aluminium toxicity for the following reasons: i) renal excretion of the element is impaired, ii) dialysate is a source of additional aluminium, and iii) aluminium hydroxide is often used as a phosphate binder. Aluminium accumulates in the bone, liver, spleen, brain, muscles, heart and parathyroid glands. Aluminium toxicity produces two main clinical patterns:

1) dialysis dementia, characterized by personality change, dyspraxia, speech disturbance, myoclonic jerks and global dementia.
2) aluminium bone disease, characterized by bone pain, diffuse demineralization and secondary fractures. Biochemically, serum calcium levels are normal or raised and serum PTH undetectable.

Diagnosis is made by measurement of serum aluminium levels, though these tend to reflect recent exposure and the rise in serum aluminium level during a desferrioxamine infusion provides more useful information. Bone biopsy remains the definitive diagnostic test.

95B a) The cerebellum.

b) The combination of polycythaemia and cerebellar signs suggests a diagnosis of von Hippel–Lindau syndrome. The syndrome is inherited in an autosomal dominant fashion. Haemangioblastoma develop throughout the central nervous system but show a predilection for the cerebellum. Von Hippel–Lindau syndrome is one of the recognized causes of ectopic erythropoietin production. Other recognized features include i) cysts affecting the kidney, liver and pancreas, ii) renal cell carcinoma, and iii) phaeochromocytoma.

96 a) The biochemical picture is one of a **high anion gap metabolic acidosis**. In the context of the given history the likely cause is **lactic acidosis** subsequent to an inferior myocardial infarction and shock.

The anion gap is an estimation of the total unmeasured plasma anions which in association with HCO_3^- and Cl^- balance plasma cations, which are predominately Na^+ and K^+ (also Mg^{2+} and Ca^{2+}).

The unmeasured plasma anions include proteins, organic acids, Po_4^{2-} and SO_4^{2-}.

For simplicity:

Anion gap = (Na mmol/l + K mmol/l) − (Cl mmol/l + HCO_3 mmol/l).
Anion gap normal range 7–17

In the above example, anion gap = 28 mmol/l.
Measurement of plasma lactate (normally less than 2 mmol/l) would confirm the diagnosis. Measurement of arterial blood gases and pH may be useful in patients of this sort.
Causes of lactic acidosis include:

1) Shock
2) Infection
3) Diabetes mellitus
4) Renal failure
5) Liver failure
6) Drugs, e.g. biguanides – phenformin and metformin, and alcohol
7) Congenital causes e.g. glucose-6-phosphate dehydrogenase deficiency.

97 a) This M-mode clearly cuts across the mitral valve. **Rheumatic fever** is the only common cause of mitral stenosis.

b) Structure A is the intraventricular septum. Right ventricle is above and left ventricle below the line.

c) The 2 leaflets of the mitral valve separate in diastole; their echo signal is normally a sharp single line each, and they move in opposite directions. B is the posterior leaflet and is
i) thickened, and ii) moves anteriorly in diastole (i.e. upwards). This is characteristic of mitral stenosis. In addition the normal pattern of movement of the leaflets is to drift together in mid-diastole and to re-open with atrial contraction. When the left atrial pressure is high they remain open at the limit of their excursion at all times, as shown here.

d) With a mobile stenosed valve, mitral valve opening can be heard as an early diastolic opening snap. This occurs at line C.

98 a) The man has presented with an acute febrile illness characterized by gastrointestinal and respiratory symptoms, unexplained confusion, mild hepatitis, hyponatraemia, hypocalcaemia and relative hypophosphataemia. The most likely diagnosis is **Legionella pneumonia**. Infection with *M pneumoniae* or an ornithosis may have similar clinical features but would not be expected to produce such a low sodium and calcium.

Legionella occurs sporadically or in epidemics. The natural habitat of *Legionella* species is fresh water; a wide temperature (5–65°C) and pH range (5.5–8.2) is acceptable. Water storage systems such as airconditioning apparatus, cooling towers and hospital hot water supplies have all been implicated as sources in a variety of epidemics.

Legionnaires' disease typically affects people between 40 and 70 years. There is a high incidence among transplant and other immunosuppressed patients. Abdominal symptoms may dominate the clinical presentation, including pain, diarrhoea and distension; rarely, peritonitis and pancreatitis occur. An enlarged liver and abnormal liver function tests are common. The pneumonia is typically widespread and may heal with fibrosis. In addition to confusion and hallucinations, ataxia, peripheral neuropathy and memory defects may occur. Hyponatraemia, hypocalcaemia, hypophosphataemia and lymphopenia are commonly seen. Haematuria occurs commonly; renal failure is rare. Pericarditis, myocarditis and endocarditis are rare.

b) Investigations should include serology for legionella, mycoplasma, and chlamydia. A bronchoscopy should be performed to obtain material for culture and microscopy (if the condition and pO_2 of the patient permit).

Antibodies start to appear 5–10 days after the onset of symptoms; for definite serological confirmation of legionella infection, comparison of acute and convalescent sera is required. A single sample with a titre of 1/250 or greater is, however, highly suggestive. Culture of the organism requires special conditions and selective media; the organism grows slowly so that 2–3 weeks may be required to detect the organism in this way. The organism may be seen on microscopy using silver stains or immunofluorescence.

c) Treatment is either with erythromycin or rifampicin. The prognosis is related to the patient's age, the severity of the pneumonia and the existence of any concomitant disease. Symptoms of poor memory and general irritability may persist for months following recover.

Chlorination and filtration of water supplies will eliminate the organism.

99 a) The most likely diagnosis is **bacterial endocarditis**.

b) Investigations should include i) serial cultures of blood and urine, ii) an echocardiogram, and iii) angiography of her left iliac artery. The upper abdominal pain, spleen tenderness and wedge defects are splenic infarcts. The pulsatile left iliac fossa mass is a mycotic aneurysm. The neurological symptoms result from emboli.

In adults nearly a third of cases of infective endocarditis develop on a previously normal valve, and another third occur in patients with mitral valve prolapse. A minority of patients who develop infective endocarditis have a previous history of serious valve disease, e.g. rheumatic fever. Cerebral emboli occur in nearly 20% of cases, typically in the middle cerebral artery territory. The formation of a cerebral mycotic aneurysm is particularly ominous since they have a high chance of rupturing, causing a subarachnoid haemorrhage or intraventricular haemorrhage.

The clinical features of infective endocarditis include fever, evidence of an acute phase response, polyclonal activation of B-cells producing raised rheumatoid factors and a false positive VDRL, petechial haemorrhages, splinter haemorrhages, Osler's nodes (pulp of the finger), Janeway lesions (on the thenar and hypothenar eminence), Roth spots (retinal infarcts), conjunctival haemorrhages, splenomegaly, and in long-standing cases, clubbing. Emboli may affect any organ. Renal lesions include both emboli and glomerulonephritis. Effects on the nervous system reflect embolic phenomena. In chronic cases a normochromic normocytic anaemia develops. The WBC may be raised, normal or in severe cases depressed.

In 90% of cases the organism is grown from blood culture; previous antibiotic administration or unusual organisms account for most of the exceptions. Both *Coxiella burnetti* and mycoplasma may cause endocarditis and can be detected serologically.

The principles of treatment are sterilization of the valve using appropriate antibiotics (usually given for six weeks) followed by surgery if the valve is badly damaged. Infection with organisms such as *Staphyloccocus aureus* or *Streptococcus pneumoniae* which are characterized by rapid tissue destruction, fungal endocarditis, patients with aortic root infection, and patients with prosthetic valves should be considered for early surgery.

100 a) Myasthaenia gravis. On examination muscle weakness may not be apparent unless strength is examined repeatedly.

b) i) Fatiguability may be demonstrated electrically by repetitive supramaximal stimulation of a suitable peripheral nerve while recording the muscle group evoked potential.

  ii) The fatiguability of the affected muscles may be temporarily corrected by edrophonium (Tensilon test).

  iii) The disease may be confirmed by detecting antibodies to acetylcholine receptors.

  iv) X-ray thoracic inlet

  v) CT scan of the neck and chest

  vi) Thyroid function tests

  vii) Autoantibody profile.

The muscles most often affected are ocular and shoulder girdle. However the muscles of respiration and proximal lower limbs may also be involved early. Breathlessness may develop very quickly and may cause sudden death. Bulbar involvement causes swallowing problems, slurred speech and difficulty chewing. External ocular muscle weakness is often asymmetrical and if a single muscle is affected may mimic a cranial nerve palsy. Pupillary reflexes are always normal. Mild ptosis and weak facial muscles may give the patient a 'snarl' or a depressed look. Eventually muscles of the neck and trunk become involved. Thymic enlargement may be seen in approximately 15% of cases, especially in young patients. In 25% of cases there is evidence of local invasion but not distal spread.

The disease is autoimmune in origin and may be associated with other diseases such as systemic lupus erythematosus, thyrotoxicosis and diabetes mellitus. Thyrotoxicosis may worsen symptoms and signs. Antibodies against acetylcholine receptors on the postsynaptic membrane have a pathogenic role.

Initial treatment is with steroids with or without azathioprine; after improvement has occurred thymectomy should be performed. The benefit of thymectomy cannot be predicted; therefore all cases with generalized disease or thymoma irrespective of age or sex should be offered the operation. Plasmapheresis by removing antibody is a useful short-term measure in severe cases. Anticholinesterase drugs such as pyridostigmine are useful in improving muscle strength.

101 a) The normal left ventricular cavity at end diastole is less than 5.5 cm across; there is therefore cavity dilatation present.
b) 'A' is a sound occurring immediately after the QRS complex of the ECG and must therefore be the first heart sound.
c) The signal occurs in the phase preceding the first heart sound and must be diastolic. The doppler signal is above the centre line which corresponds to blood flowing towards the transducer at the apex.
d) Diastolic flow across the aortic valve towards the apex can only be regurgitation. The left ventricular cavity enlargement is therefore secondary to aortic incompetence.

102 a) The most likely diagnosis is **normal pressure hydrocephalus** which is characterized by amnesia (often with psychomotor retardation), gait apraxia and urinary incontinence. There are generally few cortical features such as dysphasia or apraxia, unlike Alzheimer's disease. The onset is typically insidious but may be rapid. There is dilatation of the cerebral ventricles caused by subarachnoid obstruction but normal CSF pressure is recorded if a lumbar puncture is performed.
The syndrome has been observed following head injury, subarachnoid haemorrhage, intracranial surgery, cerebrovascular disease and meningoencephalitis, and in association with lesions which obstruct the third ventricle such as gliomas, cerebellar haemangioblastomas, aqueduct stenosis, third ventricular cysts, and aberrant blood vessels. In 50% of cases there is no clear cause. There is impaired outflow and resorption of CSF; this dilates the ventricles, stretches the periventricular pathways, reduces cerebral blood flow and causes oedema of the periventricular substance. Positron-emission tomography has demonstrated generalized disturbances of cerebral metabolism in normal pressure hydrocephalus as distinct from degenerative diseases.
b) CSF diversion procedures in selected patients can completely reverse the abnormalities (generally ventriculoatrial or ventriculo-peritoneal shunts). It is important to distinguish normal pressure hydrocephalus from the passive ventricular enlargement secondary to cerebral atrophy, which will not benefit from a shunt procedure. CT scanning and intracranial pressure measurement are useful – lack of cortical atrophy and the presence of frontal white matter and periventricular lucency favour normal pressure hydrocephalus. CSF diversion may be complicated by shunt infection, subdural haematomas, epilepsy, and malfunction.

103 a) He has a reduced peak flow, mild hypoxia, and a partially-compensated respiratory alkalosis. These results are consistent with acute asthma. Treatment is a high inspired pO_2, bronchodilators (nebulizer or intravenous) and intravenous hydrocortisone. A chest X-ray should be obtained to exclude a concomitant pneumothorax and pneumonia. The response to treatment must be monitored by reassessing his vital signs, the peak flow and blood gases after 1–2 hours.

b) The patient has become more hypoxic and has developed a respiratory acidosis. This is consistent with alveolar hypoventilation. The most important diagnosis to exclude is a pneumothorax. Other causes are impaired respiratory drive (drugs), pneumonia, a collapsed lung (obstruction of a bronchus), and patient exhaustion. Mechanical ventilation should be considered urgently if an easily-reversible cause is not rapidly identified and further deterioration occurs.

104 a) B is a murmur on the phonocardiogram which can be seen from the ECG to be systolic.

b) The aortic root is full of echos during both systole and diastole. This is due to distortion of the aortic valve. B is therefore an aortic ejection murmur.

c) The structure behind the aortic root is the left atrium. This should not exceed 4.5 cm in diameter. It is thus enlarged according to the 1 cm markers.

d) There is mitral valve disease. There are two reasons from the echocardiogram shown:
  i) Rheumatic aortic valve disease never occurs in the absence of mitral valve involvement.
  ii) Gross left atrial enlargement (7.5 cm) strongly suggests mitral valve disease.

Answer to question 105

105 a) The most likely diagnosis is **cystic fibrosis**. The young boy has evidence of malabsorption, chronic respiratory symptoms, a dilated right colon, and is small for his age.

b) Investigations should include a sweat test – the characteristic defect is that secretions contain too little water relative to the protein and electrolyte content, causing mucoviscidosis. A sodium content above 100 mmol/l is consistent with the diagnosis. Other investigations include an assessment of pancreatic function: plasma trypsin and amylase are reduced in chronic pancreatic disease because of loss of cell numbers; an oral glucose tolerance test is useful to assess endocrine pancreatic function. Direct assessment of the pancreas requires measurement of enzymes and bicarbonate in a duodenal aspirate before and after a test meal (the Lundh test), such tests are difficult to perform.

Cystic fibrosis is an autosomal recessive condition, characterized by abnormal exocrine secretion. The major clinical features include chronic pulmonary disease, pancreatic dysfunction resulting in malabsorption, poor growth and diabetes mellitus. The most important problems are respiratory: recurrent bronchiolar obstruction causes bronchiectasis, atelectasis and chronic infection which gradually destroys lung function, ultimately leading to pulmonary insufficiency, and cor pulmonale. Allergic bronchopulmonary aspergillosis is common. The lungs often become colonized by *Staphylococcus pyogenes* and *Pseudomonas aeruginosa*. Hypoplasia of the gall bladder occurs and there is an increased tendency to form gallstones; blockage of bile ducts leads to pericholangitis, periportal fibrosis and biliary cirrhosis. Intestinal problems are related to the secretion of abnormal amounts of viscid mucus and include meconium ileus, intestinal obstruction and reduced transit in the distal bowel.

Treatment is partially successful so that patients now regularly reach adulthood. Physiotherapy and replacement of pancreatic enzymes are the two principal measures. Immunization and the rapid use of antibiotics help to minimize pulmonary damage. Ranitidine is helpful in decreasing the acid digestion of pancreatic enzymes. Genetic counselling should be offered to the parents and other unaffected siblings; prenatal diagnosis is now available.

106 a) The man has progressive breathlessness, without evidence of heart failure or obstructive airways disease, and associated with a positive ANA, latex and raised immunoglobulins (high total protein). The most likely diagnosis is **cryptogenic fibrosing alveolitis.** He also has a mild biochemical hepatitis, seen in 10 % of cryptogenic fibrosing alveolitis cases. The raised urea is likely to be caused by diuretics. Since his symptoms had begun before the prescription of amiodarone this is unlikely to have been the original trigger. The main differential diagnoses to consider are:

1) Lung fibrosis associated with a connective tissue disease or vasculitis
2) Extrinsic allergic alveolitis – exposure to organic dusts
3) Bronchiectasis
4) Left sided heart failure
5) Sarcoidosis
6) Lymphangitis carcinomatosa
7) Pulmonary embolism
8) Industrial lung diseases.

b) Investigations should include pulmonary function tests, including TLCO and KCO estimation to demonstrate lung restriction and reduced gas transfer. A lung biopsy, either via a bronchoscope or an open lung biopsy, to establish a histological diagnosis and provide prognostic information. If these results were normal or the lung biopsy showed granulomas then a Kveim test and serum angiotensin-converting enzyme estimation to exclude sarcoidosis should be obtained. Finally a right heart catheter study to measure pulmonary artery pressure should be performed.

The histological features of cryptogenic fibrosing alveolitis include (i) cellular infiltration and fibrosis of the lung parenchyma and (ii) desquamation of altered type II pneumocytes and macrophages into the alveolar space. The process is patchy and individuals may have predominantly one or the other histological type. As the disease progresses fibrosis in the alveolar walls impairs gas transfer and disrupts the pulmonary vasculature; in addition there is collapse of small parts of the lung, leading to loss of functioning bronchoalveolar units. A 'loss of units pattern' is sometimes seen in mild cases, when lung restriction and loss of volume is accompanied by relative preservation of the corrected transfer factor (KCO). The histology of lung fibrosis in CFA and that seen with connective tissue diseases are similar.

There is an association of lung fibrosis with the organ-specific autoimmune diseases such as autoimmune thyroid disease and chronic active hepatitis.

107 a)   i) Right bundle branch block
      ii) Left axis deviation
      iii) First degree heart block.
b) Left axis deviation is most commonly caused by left anterior hemifascicular block. The ventricular mass is depolarized from impulses generated at the sinuatrial node, and there is conduction delay to atrioventricular nodal depolarization. The left posterior hemifascicle is the only connection between the node and the ventricular mass.

c) Syncope is evidence of the intermittent failure of left posterior hemifascicle conduction and therefore complete atrioventricular block. This is an indication of permanent pacing.

108 a) This lady has presented with pulmonary hypertension and right-sided heart failure. Pulmonary hypertension rarely occurs independently and normally the symptoms and signs of the primary causative disease predominate. In the absence of other causes the differential diagnosis in a young female lies between **primary pulmonary hypertension** and **chronic pulmonary emboli**.

Very small pulmonary emboli (microemboli) cause few or no symptoms. Repeated emboli over several months result in the development of pulmonary hypertension. A proportion of these cases are associated with pregnancy (usually following) or the oral contraceptive pill. Emboli from trophoblastic or breast tumours may rarely cause pulmonary hypertension. The diagnosis is made when asymmetric occlusions of pulmonary arteries can be demonstrated at angiography. Generally patients have an angiographic appearance identical to primary pulmonary hypertension; in such cases if no source of multiple emboli is apparent a diagnosis of primary pulmonary hypertension is made.

b) The essential investigation is cardiac catheterization, to i) confirm pulmonary hypertension and assess the right heart function; ii) to measure the wedge pressure and exclude mitral stenosis and other left heart causes of pulmonary hypertension; iii) by measuring the oxygen content assess or exclude a significant right-to-left shunt; iv) perform a pulmonary angiogram. Pulmonary angiography is rarely able to distinguish between microembolic disease and primary pulmonary hypertension.

Definitive treatment of primary pulmonary hypertension is heart–lung transplantation. If detected early, microembolic disease may be treated by anticoagulation.

109A **a)** The blood gases are consistent with **chronic mild alveolar hypoventilation**, slightly reduced pO_2, a raised pCO_2 and a compensated respiratory acidosis. This lady is a typical 'Pickwickian'. This is the label given to patients with normal mechanical ventilatory function who underbreathe. There are three factors associated with the syndrome: i) obesity, ii) mild obstructive airways disease and smoking, and iii) reduced central drive to breathe i.e. a reduced sensitivity to pCO_2.

Investigations include full pulmonary function tests, and sleep studies, i.e. monitoring of blood gases at night, since the degree of hypoventilation increases during sleep and apnoeic episodes may be observed.

b) Treatment is weight reduction, stopping smoking, and using nasal cannulae with compressed air at night to increase ventilation and reduce the number of apnoeic episodes. Long term complications of the syndrome include cor pulmonale and polycythaemia.

109B **a)** **An elevated serum creatinine subsequent to the trimethoprim**; the normal urea makes a more sinister explanation unlikely. Trimethoprim competes with creatinine for excretion by the distal convoluted tubule.

Note: there are a number of circumstances in which either the serum urea or creatinine concentration may be disproportionately increased:

Urea > Creatinine:	Creatinine > Urea:
Dehydration/pre-renal failure	Liver disease
Gastrointestinal haemorrhage	Trimethoprim/Septrin
Acute-on-chronic renal failure	Rhabdomyolysis
Corticosteroids	Dialysis
Tetracyclines	Racial – negros
Infection	Pregnancy
Post surgery	Vomiting

110 a) Tuberculous meningitis.
Adult tuberculous meningitis often has a gradual onset and may present with vague symptoms of malaise, loss of appetite, intellectual and personality changes, fever and headaches. Symptoms of meningism may be mild. As the disease progresses cranial nerve palsies or strokes may occur. The diagnosis is suggested by the CSF findings of a raised lymphocyte count despite evidence of a bloody tap, an elevated protein and a reduced glucose level. Only rarely are acid-fast bacilli seen on the ZN stains of the CSF.

b) The deterioration was caused by a cerebrovascular accident, the result of tuberculous endarteritis. Other possible causes to consider are metabolic disturbance such as hyponatraemia or the development of an obstructive hydrocephalus caused by granulomas reducing the flow of CSF.
Note: CSF findings would also be consistent with a partially-treated bacterial infection (history of antibiotics). However the duration of the illness and the complication of a cerebrovascular accident are against this.

111A a) At this stage she fulfils the criteria for a diagnosis of **benign paraproteinaemia.**
These are:
1) A relatively low concentration of paraprotein (<20 g/l)
2) Absence of Bence-Jones protein
3) Absence of immune paresis
4) A normal skeletal survey
5) A normal percentage of plasma cells in the bone marrow (<4%); occasionally the percentage is greater than 4% but definitely less than 10%
6) Maintenance of a constant level of paraprotein over a period of time.

Benign paraproteinaemia may be found in the normal healthy adult population with a frequency of up to 1% and this increases to 3% in those over 70 years of age. It may also be found in hospitalized patients suffering from a wide range of non-lymphoproliferative disorders, e.g. liver disease, connective tissue disease and neoplasia of the gut and lung.

b) Regular outpatient follow up is required to monitor the paraprotein levels and to ensure that a malignant paraprotein does not develop. Bone marrow, skeletal survey and Bence-Jones protein estimation should be repeated if there is suspicion of malignant transformation.

111B **a) Cushing's syndrome due to ectopic ACTH production.**
Ectopic ACTH production usually presents with the metabolic features of steroid excess. These are hypertension, diabetes, muscle weakness and a hypokalaemic metabolic alkalosis. In addition, marked pigmentation may occur.
   b) i) Chest X-ray. Oat cell carcinoma of the bronchus is the likely source in a smoker. Other potential sites include pancreas, thymus, thyroid and breast or carcinoid tumours.
   ii) Plasma ACTH level. Typically, very high levels are associated with ectopic ACTH production (>200 ng/l) and accompany high plasma cortisol levels (>1000 nmol/l).

112 **a) Multiple myeloma with a serum IgG paraprotein.**
The diagnosis may be confirmed by i) examining the urine for the presence of Bence-Jones protein which is present in 66% of cases, ii) bone marrow examination to show an increased percentage of plasma cells (>10%), and iii) skeletal survey to show osteolytic areas, which are present in 60% of cases.
   b) i) Clinically the patient is nephrotic and this would account for the oedema and exertional dyspnoea. Nephrotic syndrome is a common consequence of renal amyloid. The diagnosis may be confirmed by renal biopsy.
   ii) In addition the ECG changes suggest the possibility of cardiac amyloid. This typically produces a restrictive cardiomyopathy – a common cause of death in these patients. Cardiac amyloid often presents with oedema, shortness of breath and angina. The echocardiographic appearance is often diagnostic, with increased thickness of right and left ventricular walls, decreased amplitude of wall excursion and the characteristic 'granular sparkle'. Endomyocardial biopsy confirms the diagnosis.
The clinical signs and symptoms of amyloid may precede the diagnosis of an underlying immune dyscrasia. Systemic AL amyloid may complicate any B-cell dyscrasia, e.g. multiple myeloma, macroglobulinaemia, lymphoma and benign monoclonal gammopathy. Overall AL amyloid complicates 15% of cases of multiple myeloma. Other clinical features include carpal tunnel syndrome (this patient complains of median nerve compression), peripheral and autonomic neuropathy, macroglossia, gut involvement with malabsorption/haemorrhage/perforation, hepatomegaly, hyposplenism, non-thrombocytopenic purpura, arthropathy and bleeding diathesis – factor IX and X deficiency.

113 **a)** **Churg–Strauss syndrome.**

b) Churg–Strauss syndrome is a medium-vessel granulomatous vasculitis characterized by a triad of i) late onset asthma with or without allergic rhinitis, ii) a fluctuating eosinophilia, and iii) an extrapulmonary vasculitis involving 2 or more organs, e.g. the peripheral nervous system, skin, or kidney. The condition characteristically responds well to steroids.

c) i) Interstitial nephritis secondary to antibiotic therapy.

ii) Cholesterol emboli – occur in arteriopaths and may be associated with an eosinophilia and occasionally a transiently low C3.

114A **a)** **Inappropriate antidiuretic hormone secretion** with hyponatraemia, hypouricaemia, and inappropriately high urinary sodium excretion and urinary (cf plasma) osmolality. The smoking history suggests the possibility of an underlying bronchial carcinoma.

b) Increased urate clearance – not a dilutional effect!

c) i) Establish and treat the underlying cause
ii) Fluid restriction
iii) Demethylchlortetracycline – antagonizes the effects of antidiuretic hormone secretion on the distal tubules.

Causes of true inappropriate antidiuretic hormone secretion include

1) Malignancy – bronchial (small cell carcinoma), pancreas, lymphoma
2) CNS – head injury, meningitis, raised intracranial pressure, Guillain–Barré
3) Chest – infection, intermittent positive pressure ventilation
4) Drugs – chlorpropamide, cyclophosphamide, carbamazepine, vincristine, opiates, amitriptyline
5) Miscellaneous – acute intermittent porphyria, schizophrenia.

114B **a) Measurement of plasma lipids.** The patient has
pseudohyponatraemia due to nephrotic syndrome and
secondary hyperlipidaemia. The clues to this are, firstly the
normal measured plasma osmolality (cf the calculated
osmolality of $2 \times ([Na^+] + [K^+]) + [Ur] + [Gl] = 254$), the low
albumin and nephrotic range proteinuria.

Plasma sodium is measured in the aqueous phase and a
false low reading is not uncommon in hyperlipidaemic states
such as the nephrotic syndrome. More rarely, a raised serum
protein e.g. with a paraprotein, may give a milder
pseudohyponatraemia.

Note: nephrotic syndrome is associated with raised levels of
cholesterol (LDL) and when hypoalbuminaemia is severe, with
elevated levels of triglyceride (VLDL). Chronic renal failure *per
se* is associated with hypertriglyceridaemia.

115 **a)** There are two pacing spikes for each QRS complex: one
precedes the P-wave and is therefore generated by an atrial
pacing lead. The second precedes the QRS and is generated
by a ventricular lead.

Atrial pacing will be inhibited by a native P-wave. Absence
of native P-waves indicates sinus node disease.

If the AV node was functioning, the P-waves generated by
the atrial pacing lead would cause a normal QRS complex.
This does not happen, and in the absence of a normal QRS
complex there is a paced beat (left bundle branch block
morphology) – this indicates failure of atrioventricular
conduction.

116 a) 400 mmol. {Calculated from: ⅓ body weight (approx. vol of distribution) × base excess}

b) Ethylene glycol poisoning. Recognized complications include cardiac failure and arrhythmias, pulmonary failure and acute renal failure which may complicate oxalate deposition.

c) i) Removal of ethylene glycol by haemodialysis; ii) treatment of acidosis; iii) ethanol infusion.

The causes of high anion gap acidosis are legion and include all causes of lactic acidosis. In the context of an overdose, consideration should be given to aspirin, paracetamol, methanol and ethylene glycol toxicity.

Ethylene glycol (antifreeze) is metabolized to oxalate, via glycoaldehyde and glycollate. The oxalate precipitates in the urine as calcium oxalate, causing crystalluria. Typically, it takes 12 hours from ingestion for symptoms to develop, somewhat less than is the case for methanol. Methanol toxicity is due to metabolism to the toxic metabolite formate and is dominated clinically by visual symptoms.

Optimum treatment, for both methanol and ethylene glycol toxicity, consists of bicarbonate dialysis to remove the toxin and treat the acidosis, and an ethanol infusion. Ethanol is preferentially metabolized by alcohol dehydrogenase, for which both methanol and ethylene glycol are substrates, thus preventing the generation of toxic metabolites.

117 a) Renal artery stenosis due to fibromuscular dysplasia.

b) The disease is bilateral – in unilateral disease, one would expect an increased renal vein renin from the affected kidney, with suppression of the unaffected kidney.

c) In a young woman fibromuscular dysplasia is the most likely cause. The treatment of choice is percutaneous angioplasty in this case. Atheromatous disease in older patients may require surgery.

d) Following renal artery angioplasty or surgical bypass, a considerable diuresis may occur. Careful monitoring and rehydration are needed, and the patient's antihypertensive therapy may require modification.

118 a) Multiple myeloma complicated by proximal renal tubular acidosis (type II).
Investigations show a normochromic normocytic anaemia, an elevated ESR, hypercalcaemia, and an elevated alkaline phosphatase (note: alkaline phosphatase is only elevated when pathological fracture occurs: the patient presents with back pain). The hyperchloraemic hypokalaemic metabolic acidosis and glycosuria in the presence of a normal plasma glucose are typical of proximal renal tubular acidosis. Other recognized features of proximal renal tubular acidosis include aminoaciduria, and increased urate and phosphate clearance with concomitant hypouricaemia and hypophosphataemia phosphataemia – the Fanconi syndrome.

In type II renal tubular acidosis, the proximal tubules fail in their normal function of reabsorption of bicarbonate (HCO_3-) – normally approximately 85% of the filtered bicarbonate load. There is therefore an increased delivery of bicarbonate to the distal tubule which is unable to reabsorb the excess, resulting in bicarbonaturia. As the serum bicarbonate falls, so does the proximal tubular bicarbonate concentration until it is below the T_{max} for bicarbonate, at which point bicarbonaturia ceases and net acid production and excretion are balanced. It is because of this that, unlike RTA type I, additional buffering from bone is not required and therefore osteomalacia and hypercalciuria do not occur. Sodium is the obligate cation lost with bicarbonate in the urine and the resulting volume depletion leads to stimulation of the renin–angiotensin–aldosterone pathway and hence to hypokalaemia. Hyperchloraemia is a result of eventual compensatory enhanced sodium and chloride reabsorption in response to hypovolaemia.

b) The appropriately low urine pH in this patient is explained by the fact that this was an early morning sample. Low urine flow at this time allows adequate acidification by a normal distal tubule.

c) i) To confirm the diagnosis of multiple myeloma: skeletal survey, bone marrow examination, measurement of serum immunoglobulins, protein electrophoresis and urine examination for Bence-Jones protein; ii) to confirm the diagnosis of proximal renal tubular acidosis: bicarbonate loading test. In a HCO_3- loading test, the T_{max} for HCO_3- (tubular maximal reabsorption of HCO_3-) is soon exceeded and a fractional HCO_3- excretion of greater than 15% of the filtered load occurs in cases of proximal renal tubular acidosis (compared with approximately 5% in distal renal tubular acidosis).

d) Albumin – aminoacids and Bence-Jones proteins do not register on urinary dipsticks.

119 a) i) Renal ultrasound scan or CT scan
ii) Renal angiography.
The patient has developed a **renal cell carcinoma
(hypernephroma)**. There is an increased incidence of renal cell
carcinoma in adult polycystic disease.
In a patient with polycystic kidneys it is easy to overlook the
possibility of renal cell carcinoma as the classic triad of loin
pain, haematuria and a mass may all be attributed to the
polycystic kidneys *per se*. The principal clue in this patient's
case is the hypercalcaemia, which is best explained as ectopic
production of a PTH-like peptide – one of several paraneoplastic
manifestations of a hypernephroma.
The increased alkaline phosphatase is one of several
recognized abnormalities of liver function associated with renal
cell carcinomas. The others include increased bilirubin and
alpha-2 globulin concentrations, and a prolonged prothrombin
time.

b) The haemoglobin concentration is inappropriately high for
the degree of renal failure: i) adult polycystic kidney disease *per
se* is associated with increased erythropoietin production, which
tends to maintain the haemoglobin concentration; ii) dehydration
secondary to the hypercalcaemia. The serum urea is
disproportionately elevated compared with the serum creatinine;
iii) polycythaemia due to erythropoietin excretion is a rare
paraneoplastic complication of hypernephromas.

c) None. All patients with chronic renal failure will retain PTH
C-terminal and this has no biological significance. The most
appropriate assay for PTH in chronic renal failure is an
N-terminal or whole molecule assay. This will not, however,
except in rare circumstances, detect a paraneoplastic PTH-like
peptide.

120 a) The bicarbonate concentration is 14.5 mmol/l.

Anion gap = {[Na⁺] + [K⁺]} − {[Cl⁻] + [HCO₃⁻]}

$$\text{Anion gap} = \{[Na^+] + [K^+]\} - \{[Cl^-] + [HCO_3^-]\}$$

b) Renal tubular acidosis type I – the biochemical picture of a hyperchloraemic hypokalaemic acidosis with a normal anion gap is typical. The patient is unable to acidify the urine despite having a metabolic acidosis. Nephrocalcinosis and renal colic are well-recognized complications of distal renal tubule acidosis and accounts for the loin pain.
Note: An NH_4Cl loading test is only of use if the patient does not have a systemic acidosis. Conversely the patient does not have renal tubule acidosis if the pH of the urine is less than 5.5.

Causes of distal and proximal renal tubular acidosis include:

Distal renal tubular acidosis	Proximal renal tubular acidosis
Primary	Primary
Hereditary	Hereditary
Acquired	Wilson's disease
Autoimmune disease	Galactosaemia
Hypergammaglobulinaemia	Cystinosis
Sjøgren's disease	Lowe's syndrome
Chronic active hepatitis	Fructose intolerance
Nephrocalcinosis	Autoimmune disease
Hyperparathyroidism	Sjøgren's syndrome
Vitamin D intoxication	Dysproteinaemic states
Medullary sponge kidney	Multiple myeloma
Idiopathic hypercalciuria	Drugs
Tubulo-interstitial disease	Acetazolamide
Obstructive uropathy	Lead
Chronic pyelonephritis	Tetracyclines
Sickle cell disease	Miscellaneous
Drugs	Hypocalcaemia
Analgesic nephropathy	Hyperparathyroidism
Lithium	Amyloid
Amphotericin	Nephrotic syndrome

121 a) Epigastric discomfort; vomiting; nausea; sweating and hyperpyrexia; irritability, tinnitus, deafness, tremor; increased respiratory rate (pulmonary oedema); dehydration; hypokalaemia; bruising/purpura – secondary to hypoprothrombinaemia.

b) Both acid–base and fluid/electrolyte disturbances occur: initially, respiratory alkalosis; later, metabolic acidosis; hyper- or hypoglycaemia may occur.

c) Initial respiratory alkalosis is due to direct stimulation of the respiratory centre by salicylate. To compensate for this bicarbonate is secreted in the urine, with loss of Na, K and water. The reduction in bicarbonate reduces the buffering capacity of blood
Acidosis develops partly from the presence of salicylic acid, and partly as a result of interference with intermediary metabolism – e.g. TCA cycle inhibition results in an increase in lactate and pyruvate; stimulation of fat catabolism causes ketone body and β-hydroxybutyrate production (also starvation and dehydration); accelerated protein catabolism causes aminoacidaemia/uria.
Salicylates uncouple oxidative phosphorylation, thereby increasing oxygen utilization and carbon dioxide production; energy dissipated as heat and increased tissue glycolysis occurs. Severe dehydration can result with pre-renal renal failure.

d) 300–500 mg/l at 6 hrs: mild toxicity
500–750 mg/l: moderate
>750 mg/l: severe toxicity;
>1000 mg/l: consider haemoperfusion/dialysis

e)   i) Gastric aspiration/lavage – ipecacuanha in a child
   ii) Activated charcoal orally
   iii) Correction of dehydration with i.v. saline
   iv) Correction of hypokalaemia
   v) Correction of severe metabolic acidocis with i.v. bicarbonate
   vi) Tepid sponging
   vii) Forced alkaline diuresis if salicylate level >750 mg/l – monitor CVP. Urine pH 8–8.5
   viii) Haemodialysis or haemoperfusion
   ix) Vitamin K for hypoprothrombinaemia

122 a) The patient presents with pyrexia, a right pleural effusion and leg oedema. Investigations reveal anaemia of chronic disease, an elevated ESR, hypoalbuminaemia, increased gammaglobulins, mildly deranged liver function tests and blood cultures positive for *Streptococcus milleri*. **The clinical picture is typical of an S. milleri hepatic abscess.**
Only 50% of patients complain of abdominal pain and a similar proportion have palpable hepatomegaly. Blood cultures are positive in 50–60% of cases and the organism is grown from aspirated pus in over 90% of cases.
The diagnosis should be confirmed by hepatic ultrasound which has a sensitivity of over 90%.
Streptococcus milleri, a facultative anaerobe, accounts for over 80% of pyogenic hepatic abscesses in the UK. Sixty percent of cases are associated with underlying disease, e.g. cholangitis, appendicitis, diverticulitis, Crohn's disease, or carcinoma of the colon. The incidence is highest in males and occurs more commonly in diabetics and alcoholics.

b) Management in this case is straightforward and consists of drainage of the abscess, and antibiotics. In cases where blood cultures are negative, it is essential to exclude hydatid and amoebic causes of hepatic abscess (by the appropriate serological tests, stool examination and CT scan) prior to drainage. Drainage may be percutaneous or open.
Streptococcus milleri is penicillin-sensitive and 2–6 weeks' therapy with a combination of penicillin and gentamicin is recommended.

123 a) Lateral medullary syndrome of Wallenberg.

b) Patients have dysphagia and dysarthia, ipsilateral cerebellar signs, ipsilateral Horner's syndrome, ipsilateral reduction in pin prick and temperature in the face, and contralateral pin prick and temperature loss in the limbs.

c) i) In the medulla (laterally placed)
ii) the posterior inferior cerebellar artery, though in 25% of cases the syndrome arises from vertebral artery occlusion.

d) Dysphagia/dysarthria – IXth and Xth nuclei. Vomiting – Nucleus ambiguus; hiccough – reticular formation; vertigo – vestibular nuclei; cerebellar ataxia of the limbs on the side of the lesion – inferior cerebellar peduncle; Horner's syndrome – ipsilateral – descending autonomic fibres; reduced pin prick and temperature sensation on the face on the side of the lesion – Vth nucleus; reduced pinprick and temperature sensation over the opposite limbs – lateral lemniscus (the pain/temp fibres synapse in the posterior horn, and 2nd order neurons give rise to fibres that cross in the cord, joining the contralateral spinothalamic tract, which reaches the thalamus via the lemniscus lying in a *lateral* position in the pons and medulla).

124 a) Mesangiocapillary glomerulonephritis (MCGN) type II – dense deposit disease, associated with facial lipodystrophy.

Investigations show an active urine sediment and the principal clues to the diagnosis of MCGN II are the serological picture of a low C3 and normal C4 coupled with the registrar's description of the patient, which would be consistent with the appearance of facial lipodystrophy.

Measurement of serum C3 nephritic factor (C3NeF), an antibody which results in stabilization of the alternative pathway convertase, and complement consumption, is present in up to 70% of cases.

b) Common causes of renal impairment associated with a low C3 include:

1) Systemic lupus erythematosus
2) Idiopathic MCGN type II and III
3) Post-streptococcal nephritis
4) Infective endocarditis
5) Shunt nephritis.

The other possible disorders are less likely for a number of reasons, not least because they would all be expected to activate the classical complement pathway as well as the alternative pathway, and have low levels of C4 and total haemolytic complement.

There are no features to support a diagnosis of systemic lupus erythematosus, post-streptococcal nephritis or infectious endocarditis.

C3NeF is detected in 20–30% of cases of mesangiocapillary glomerulonephritis type I; there is however no association with facial lipodystrophy.

125 a) Wenckebach phenomenon: progressive second degree atrioventricular block.

There is progressive atrioventricular delay (P–R interval) until there is one period of complete atrioventricular block, after which the cycle restarts.

126 **a) Minimal change glomerulonephritis** presenting with the nephrotic syndrome. Minimal change glomerulonephritis is most commonly idiopathic but may be associated with i) atropy, ii) drugs, e.g. aspirin and other non-steroidal anti-inflammatory agents, iii) lymphoproliferative disorders, and iv) viral infections.
b) The patient has developed renal vein thrombosis. Clinical clues to this are the deterioration in renal function, loin pain and haematuria. The history of acute shortness of breath suggests the possibility of secondary pulmonary embolism. There is a well-recognized increase in the incidence of venous thrombosis in nephrotic patients. Factors contributing to this increased risk include i) loss of fibrinolytic factors in urine – principally antithrombin III but also protein C, protein S and plasminogen, ii) increased synthesis of clotting factors – factors V, VIII and fibrinogen, iii) thrombocytosis, and iv) over-diuresis, as in this case resulting in dehydration, reducing renal blood flow and increasing viscosity.

127 **a) This is a nodal rhythm** with clear retrograde P-wave conduction, notably in V1–V3.

128 a) Guillain-Barré syndrome.

b) Lumbar puncture:
CSF Normal pressure
Raised protein (N = 45 mg/dl)
Normal cell numbers
The differential diagnosis of a raised CSF protein and normal cell count and glucose level includes spinal cord block (Froin's syndrome); intracranial tumour (commonly internal acoustic neuroma).

c) Most patients are initially managed on a general ward by urinary catheter, nasogastric feeding, and physiotherapy. It is vital to keep joints mobile and functional; pressure area care, maintenance of morale/psychological state of both patient and family are important aspects of management.

Spirometry and blood gases should be regularly monitored as rapid deterioration may require intensive care. Criteria for admission to ICU include i) severe weakness, ii) fall in vital capacity to <1.1 litres, and iii) infection and increasing hypoxia and hypercapnia. Ventilatory support often with a tracheostomy, may be required for weeks or months.

The role of immunosuppression/steroids is controversial, but plasma exchange may be beneficial.

Prognosis in Guillain-Barré – patients avoiding ventilation often recover completely, and ventilated patients may have surprisingly little residual handicap, though long-term sequelae and the need for rehabilitation are commoner in this group. Less than 5% of patients have a recurrence of the disease.

d) Miller–Fisher syndrome – external ophthalmoplegia, ataxia, areflexia
Polyneuritis cranialis – diffuse cranial nerve involvement
Chronic relapsing polyneuritis.

129 a) Acute renal failure and haemoptysis due to **antiglomerular basement membrane disease**. The differential diagnosis includes Wegener's granulomatosis, microscopic polyarteritis and systemic lupus erythematosus.
  i) Is he a smoker? Is there any history of exposure to petrol, solvents/paints? These are recognized risk factors for lung haemorrhage in anti-GBM disease; other risk factors include recent infection and pulmonary oedema.
  ii) Does he have any history of arthralgia, myalgia, rash, nasal symptoms, or jaundice? What has happened to his weight?

b) Urine microscopy evidence for an active urinary sediment; blood gases; group and save; anti-GBM assay; antineutrophil cytoplasmic antibody titre (ANCA) – elevated in cases of Wegener's granulomatosis and microscopic polyarteritis; antinuclear antibody titre (ANF); lung function tests – KCO is elevated with pulmonary haemorrhage; renal ultrasound and biopsy.

ECG changes are due to hyperkalaemia; CXR changes are due to lung haemorrhage or oedema.

c) Treatment of hyperkalaemia and fluid overload – intravenous calcium, dextrose/insulin, Ca resonium, acute dialysis.

Acutely, plasma exchange is of benefit in removing the circulating anti-GBM antibody and is of particular benefit in the treatment of lung haemorrhage. This should be combined with immunosuppressive therapy in the form of high-dose corticosteroids and cyclophosphamide, the latter being replaced after 2 months with azathioprine. Overall survival is good but the renal prognosis in anti-GBM disease is poor as the diagnosis is often late.

130A a) Chondrocalcinosis. The patient has **haemochromatosis.**
Haemochromatosis is an autosomal recessive inborn error
of metabolism which leads to a positive iron balance. Males
are affected more commonly than females and usually present
in the 4th–6th decades.
The classic triad of i) diabetes, ii) hepatomegaly and iii) the
slate-grey skin pigment (due to increased melanin deposition)
may be accompanied by hypogonadotrophic hypogonadism,
chondrocalcinosis, dilated cardiomyopathy, weakness and
weight loss.
Note: There is an increased incidence of hepatoma in
patients with cirrhosis.

b) Measure serum iron and ferritin concentrations: both will
be elevated and serum transferrin saturation will be greater
than 80%.
Measure blood glucose, which will be elevated.
Measure liver function tests.
Gonadotrophin and testosterone levels will be low.
Liver biopsy will show iron overload and the degree of
hepatic damage.
Desferrioxamine infusion will show increased urine iron
excretion.
X-ray the knees to show typical cartilage calcification.

130B a) The patient's elevated HbA1c confirms she is a **diabetic (HB
A1c** should be less than 6%).

b) Serum renin concentration is likely to be low.
The patient has impaired renal function, a hyperchloraemic,
hyperkalaemic metabolic acidosis, proteinuria and
hypertension. All these features are explicable by diabetic
nephropathy and Type IV renal tubular acidosis. Type IV renal
tubular acidosis, or hyporeninaemic hypoaldosteronism, is a
well-recognized complication of elderly, hypertensive,
chronically hyperglycaemic diabetics and is particularly likely
to develop following administration of prostaglandin
synthetase inhibitors, suggesting a causative role of
prostaglandin deficiency in the generation of this complication.
Serum renin levels are low and result in acquired
hypoaldosteronism with resulting hyperkalaemia and acidosis.

c) An arrhythmia due to the hyperkalaemia.

d) i) Hyperkalaemia *per se*, or ii) diabetic amyotrophy.

Index